SEX, DRUGS, AND THE CONTINUING SPREAD OF AIDS

Clyde B. McCoy
University of Miami

James A. Inciardi
University of Delaware

Roxbury Publishing Company

Library of Congress Cataloging-in-Publication Data

McCoy, Clyde B., 1941-
Sex, drugs, and the continuing spread of AIDS/by Clyde B. McCoy
and James A. Inciardi.
p. cm.
Includes bibliographical references and index.
ISBN 0-935732-64-0
1. AIDS (Disease)—Epidemiology. I. Inciardi, James A. II. Title.
RA644.A25M393 1994   94-13908
614.5'993—dc20   CIP

SEX, DRUGS, AND THE CONTINUING SPREAD OF AIDS

Publisher and Editor: Claude Teweles
Copy Editing: Joyce Rappaport
Line Editing: Dawn VanDercreek and Sacha Howells
Cover Design: Marnie Deacon (inspired by the work of artist
  Robert Nelson)
Typography: Synergistic Data Systems

Printed on acid-free paper in the United States of America. This
paper meets the standards for recycling of the Environmental
Protection Agency.

ISBN 0-935732-64-0

ROXBURY PUBLISHING COMPANY
P.O. Box 491044
Los Angeles, California 90049-9044
(213) 653-1068

To our daughters, Jeanene and Kristin,

whose generation must accept the challenge of HIV

and its eventual eradication.

Acknowledgements

Appreciation is extended to the following researchers, scholars, and colleagues whose comments, suggestions, and assistance at various stages of our writing were most helpful in developing the manuscript: Gary L. Albrecht, University of Illinois (Chicago); Robert S. Anwyl, Miami-Dade Community College; Sherry Deren, National Development and Research Institutes; Robert Fullilove, Columbia University; Robert S. Gossweiler, University of Delaware; Jay Johnson, University of Texas (Houston); Joseph A. Kotarba, University of Houston; Nova Lee McKernan, University of Delaware; Chancy Rawleigh, Indiana University of Pennsylvania; H. Laurence Ross, University of New Mexico; Christine Saum, University of Delaware; Paul Shapshak, University of Miami School of Medicine; Hilary L. Surratt, University of Miami School of Medicine; and others whose names are not known to us.

Clyde B. McCoy
Miami, Florida

James A. Inciardi
Key Largo, Florida

Table Of Contents

Acknowledgements iv

Preface vi
   The Continuing Spread of AIDS

Chapter One 1
   AIDS: A Strange and Deadly Epidemic

Chapter Two 29
   Contagious Desire: Sex, Drugs, Disease, and HIV

Chapter Three 67
   Bathhouses, Shooting Galleries, and Other
   Reservoirs of Infection

Chapter Four 93
   The Heterosexual Transmission of HIV

Chapter Five 123
   HIV/AIDS Prevention and Risk Reduction

Epilogue 149
   Viral Evolution and *Behavioral* Quarantine

Name Index 165

Subject Index 175

The Continuing Spread of AIDS

O f all the modern epidemic diseases, Acquired Immune Deficiency Syndrome (AIDS) is likely the most insidious, and certainly among the most feared. Like most afflictions, it can strike anyone—women and men, adults and adolescents, mothers and their infant children. But unlike other diseases, the average incubation period for AIDS may be as long as ten years—perhaps even longer. This means that a person can carry the virus for a few months to more than a decade and a half before the first symptoms appear. These symptoms may be night sweats, chronic fatigue, glandular swellings, or weight loss. During the incubation period, it is possible that those with the disease can infect others without knowing it. Once AIDS is diagnosed, the patient might live six months, a year, or three, four, five or more years. Death, however, is an eventual and virtual certainty.

Since there is no cure for AIDS, the patient must await the onset of one or more major diseases that his or her immune system will be unable to fight off—meningitis, perhaps, or pneumonia, or the feared Kaposi's sarcoma, whose purple skin lesions mark the first sign of AIDS in many people. As this unusual form of cancer develops, the lesions appear on and within the body, and the affliction is not only painful, but mutilating as well.

These factors have contributed to the sense of crisis that surrounds the AIDS epidemic. The foreboding character of the crisis tends to be heightened by the fact that many in the general population are still unwilling to believe that AIDS is *infectious* rather than *contagious*—that is, that it can be transmitted only through the exchange of bodily fluids, and not through the air or by casual contact. To this can be added the sense of isolation that the majority of persons with AIDS experience. In this respect, no one has captured the unique exile that an epidemic of this type imposes than the French novelist Albert Camus. In *The Plague*, published in 1947, Camus wrote:

There was always something missing in their lives. Hostile to the past, impatient of the present, and cheated of the future, we were much like those whom men's justice, or hatred, forces to live behind prison bars. . . . The plague had swallowed everything and everyone. No longer were there individual destinies, only a collective destiny, made of plague and the emotions shared by all. Strongest of these emotions was the sense of exile and deprivation, with all the crosscurrents of revolt and the fear set up by these.[1]

Given the media attention to AIDS and to HIV—the virus that causes AIDS—it is likely that most people in the United States have at least heard of the disease. However, other than being informed about the basic ways that AIDS is transmitted, the majority of Americans are unfamiliar with the specifics of the disease continuum. HIV, or *human immunodeficiency virus*, is a retrovirus, a type of infectious agent that had previously been identified as causing many animal diseases. HIV destroys the body's immune system, and is transmitted when virus particles or infected cells gain direct access to the bloodstream. This can occur through all forms of sexual intercourse, through using contaminated hypodermic needles and injection equipment, through blood and blood products, and through the passing of the virus from infected mothers to their unborn or newborn children. Within this context, HIV is a continuum of conditions associated with immune dysfunction, and AIDS is best described as a severe manifestation of infection with HIV.

Given the mechanisms of infection, the major transmission categories for HIV and AIDS include men who have sex with other men, persons who share injection equipment, and recipients of blood products. Also significant is the transmission of HIV to persons who have had heterosexual contacts with infected partners, and infants whose mothers are infected with HIV.

In the United States, men who have sex with men or who inject drugs represent the vast majority of known AIDS cases. Other members of the AIDS caseload reflect relatively small numbers. However, the heterosexual spread of HIV in the United States is increasing, particularly in those cities and communities where rates of injection drug use are high. Elsewhere in the world, especially in the developing nations, heterosexual spread is the major route of transmission. At issue is the extent to which heterosexual transmission will have an impact on the general escalation of AIDS. During the past decade, there have been conflicting arguments about this question. *Sex, Drugs, and the Continuing Spread of AIDS* addresses this debate. More importantly, however, the topics that follow offer readers a variety of perspectives on the nature and origins of AIDS,[2] its social dimensions and impact on people and institutions, and alternatives for reducing the continuing spread of the disease.

Much of the data reported in this book comes from our own work with drug users and other people with AIDS, and through contacts in the gay community, the street drug cultures, and the drug and AIDS treatment systems in Florida, New York, California, Delaware, Puerto Rico, and Brazil.

NOTES

1. Albert Camus, *The Plague* (New York: Alfred A. Knopf, 1947), p. 47.
2. Although Chapters One and Two of this volume provide an overview of the origins and history of AIDS, a thorough history of the epidemic is not included here. For excellent historical examinations, see Randy Shilts, *And The Band Played On: Politics, People and the AIDS Epidemic* (New York: St. Martin's Press, 1987); Jacques Leibowitch, *A Strange Virus of Unknown Origins* (New York: Ballantine Books, 1985); James Kinsella, *Covering the Plague: AIDS and the American Media* (New Brunswick, NJ: Rutgers University Press, 1989); Mirko D. Grmek, *History of AIDS: Emergence and Origin of a Modern Pandemic* (Princeton, NJ: Princeton University Press, 1990).

CHAPTER ONE

AIDS: A Strange and Deadly Epidemic

The array of bacteria, viruses, parasites, and other microbes that are sequestered in remote parts of the world likely number in the millions. Many are only partially understood by the medical community, others remain unknown to most of the world. What is eminently clear, however, is that the tropical parts of the world are quite hospitable to deadly microbes that efficiently breed to sire new diseases with unusual regularity. In some villages in West Africa, Latin America, and the Middle East, for example, it is not uncommon to see children leading their blind elders in the fields and along the roadways. With eyes full of parasitic worms and skin covered by itchy nodules, these adults suffer from *onchocerciasis*, a disease caused by a parasitic worm passed from person to person by the bite of the black fly. The parasites, which live under the skin and can grow to more than two feet in length, produce millions of microscopic offspring that eventually invade the eyes. The flies breed near fast-moving tropical streams, hence leading to the disease more commonly known as "river blindness." Few in the West have even heard of *onchocerciasis*, although the disease afflicts some 18 million people in the developing world and permanently blinds some 500,000 annually.[1]

Although river blindness is an ancient pestilence, others are newly emergent and strike both rapidly and mysteriously. A curious example in this regard was what became known as the Ebola fever virus. In 1976, the affliction swept seemingly from nowhere into the border region between Zaire and Sudan, on the banks of the Ebola River, the headstream of Central Africa's Mongala River.[2] It began when a trader from a local border village, suffering from fevers and profuse and uncontrollable bleeding, arrived at a teaching hospital for nurses in Maridi, a small town a few miles across the border into Sudan. Within days, 40 percent of the nurses had contracted the disease, transmitted by contact with their patient's blood. In Central Africa, basic supplies of disposable needles and sterile gloves were limited. Needles were used again and again, gloves were reused until they wore through, and direct and unprotected contact with blood and waste occurred when necessity demanded it.

As a blood-born disease, Ebola fever virus was also spreading rapidly through sexual intercourse and the sharing of needles in local bush hospitals. Investigations found that transmission also occurred through autopsies and ritual contact with corpses during funeral rites. The source of the virus was never determined, but after strict quarantine procedures were established, Ebola fever disappeared as rapidly as it had first materialized. During its course, however, it had infected 381 people, and was fatal in 88 percent of the cases.[3]

Across the South Atlantic in the Amazon and other tropical regions of South America, there are outbreaks of amebic and bacillary dysenteries, yellow, blackwater, and dengue fevers, as well as both malaria and cholera. And as in Central Africa, there are powerful insects and protozoa. One of these is *Rodnius prolixus*—phylum Anthropoda, class Insecta, order Hemiptera, family Reduviidae. Better known as the "assassin bug," this little creature of the equatorial bush, red and black with yellow lines down its wing cases and a stout injecting apparatus instead of a nose, is celebrated in the medical literature for one of its more offensive and disagreeable habits. Hiding during the day in cracks in the walls of human habitations, it ventures out at night for its blood meal. It bites its victims on the face or neck, and then, engorged and satiated, defecates next to the puncture.[4] There is a slight itch, and the resulting scratch pushes the droppings into the wound and thence into the bloodstream. The problem is this: those droppings carry a cargo of the microscopic protozoan parasite, *Trypanosoma cruzi*, the cause of Chagas' disease.[5] Symptoms, which begin to appear between one and 20 years after infection, include alterations of the heartbeat, heart enlargement, and a variety of glandular and nervous disorders. Like the Ebola fever virus, it can be transmitted through contact with infected blood. Transmission to newborns has occurred through blood contamination of breast milk due to nipple bleeding.[6] Chagas' disease is often fatal, and it is estimated that as many as 18 million people in the tropics are afflicted.[7]

Medications have been developed that can stem the course of river blindness; the Ebola fever virus outbreak was stopped after only a few weeks.* The risks for Chagas' disease can be reduced through insecticides and a shifting away from backland stick-and-mud home building

---

*A second outbreak of Ebola fever occurred in the Sudan in 1979, killing two-thirds of those infected. See Robin Marantz Henig, *A Dancing Matrix: Voyages Along the Viral Frontier* (New York: Alfred A. Knopf, 1993).

methods. Nevertheless, there are numerous parallels between these afflictions and AIDS, particularly in that they are unusual, incompletely understood, and are transmitted through close human contact. But AIDS is also quite different: it has no geographical restrictions, it has no cure, and the course of the disease seems to have no limits. As such, AIDS confronts everyone with a variety of concerns about risk factors and disease vectors, as well as susceptibility, contagion, and the spread of a disorder that appears to be killing virtually all of those it infects.

THE BEGINNINGS OF THE AIDS EPIDEMIC

Acquired Immune Deficiency Syndrome was first described as a new and distinct clinical entity during the late spring and early summer of 1981.[8] First, clinical investigators in Los Angeles reported five cases of *Pneumocystis carinii* pneumonia (PCP) among homosexual men to the Centers for Disease Control. None of these patients had an underlying disease that might have been associated with PCP or a history of treatment for a compromised immune system. All, however, had other clinical manifestations and laboratory evidence of immunosuppression. Second, and within a month, 26 cases of Kaposi's sarcoma (KS) were reported among homosexual men in New York and California.

When *The New York Times* first reported on these observations, the bewilderment in the medical community was clear:

> Researchers do not know the cause of the disease, let alone a successful treatment. Though several victims in California said they visited New York, doctors say indirect evidence points away from contagion. Cancer, generally, is not believed to be contagious. Investigators are considering several hypotheses, including a possible link between the cancer and past infections.[9]

What was so unusual was that prior to these reports, the appearance of both PCP and KS in populations of previously healthy young men was unprecedented. PCP is an infection caused by the parasite *P. carinii*, heretofore seen almost exclusively in cancer and transplant patients receiving immunosuppressive drugs. Prior to the age of AIDS, *Pneucystis carinii* pneumonia was one of the perhaps thousands of malevolent microorganisms that always lurked near human beings. PCP was first observed in guinea pigs and identified in 1909 and 1910 by Brazilian virologists. Three years later, physicians at the Institute Pasteur in France found that the same microbe lived quite comfortably in the lungs of Parisian sewer rats.[10] As one of the tens of thousands of creatures that exist in almost every corner of the world's inhabited terrain but easily held in check by a normally functioning immune system, *P. carinii* was identified in human lungs during World War II in Europe. In 1956, it was diagnosed in the United States for the first time among immunosuppressed patients.[11]

Kaposi's sarcoma, a cancer or tumor of the blood vessel walls, typically appears as blue-violet to brownish skin blotches. *Sarcoma* is a medical term describing a tumor that is often malignant, and Kaposi's sarcoma has been observed in a number of non-AIDS populations. It had been quite rare in the United States—occurring primarily in elderly men, usually of Mediterranean or Jewish origin. Like PCP, however, KS had also been reported among organ transplant recipients and others receiving immunosuppressive therapy. First described in 1872 by the Viennese dermatologist Moritz Kaposi as a "multiple pigmented sarcoma of the skin," it was an extremely rare malignancy for over a century in both the United States and Europe. Clinically, it appeared most frequently as a tumor of the feet and lower extremities. It was not accompanied by immune suppression, other than the expected immunological attrition associated with aging.

During the early 1960s, studies in Uganda revealed that KS was a common cancer—representing up to 9 percent of all cancers in the region. But again, no associated immunodeficiency was evident, even though a few reports of particularly aggressive cases, often in the young, were recorded. The only non-AIDS population to develop KS with parallels to current AIDS-related cases were patients receiving immunosuppressive therapy following kidney transplants. As with many AIDS patients, the cancer was often aggressive. However, KS in transplant patients often regressed completely after the withdrawal of the immunosuppressive drugs.[12]

The fact that both PCP and KS had been reported among patients receiving immunosuppressive therapy quickly led to the hypothesis that the increased occurrences of the two disorders in homosexual men were due to some underlying immune system dysfunction. This hypothesis was further supported by the incidence among homosexuals of "opportunistic infections"—infections caused by microorganisms that rarely generate disease in persons with normal immune defense mechanisms.

The presence of opportunistic infections was perplexing to the medical community. In mid-1982, for example, cases of severe illness were discovered among Haitian refugees at Miami's Jackson Memorial Hospital. Among the spectrum of diseases noticed in the group was *toxoplasmosis*,[13] a parasitical infection that can lead to lesions of the central nervous system, lungs, liver, heart, and brain. From the *T. gondii* parasite, it is distributed worldwide and affects virtually all mammalian species. Humans can acquire the organism through contaminated food or water, blood transfusions, organ transplantation, and *in utero*. Drinking contaminated water or eating uncooked meat or foods contaminated by cat feces may lead to infection. Pet cats are a well-known source of *T. gondii*, and prior to the age of AIDS the parasite lived in a latent, asymptomatic state in healthy people, or emerged as a self-limiting disease resembling mononucleosis. But in the group of Haitian refugees in Miami during 1982, and in others who would later be found to be suffering from AIDS, disease manifestation included blindness and brain dysfunction.[14]

Dr. B. H. Kean, Emeritus Professor of Tropical Medicine and Public Health at Cornell University Medical College, recently recalled a similarly perplexing incident.[15] In early 1982, at about the same time that the unexplained illness of the Haitian immigrants was being explored in Miami, one of Kean's patients complained of what appeared to be a severe case of amebic dysentery. The symptoms included cramps, nausea, and the tenacious diarrhea typically associated with visiting the tropics. Cholera was Kean's first thought, but tests found that his patient's stools were devoid of all known causes of diarrhea, and the blood studies were perfectly normal. Further investigation found the parasite *Cryptosporidium* in the patient's intestines.

Cryptosporidiosis had never been associated with human disease until the mid-1970s, when it was observed to induce severe and persistent diarrhea in a few patients with congenital immune deficiency. It had been recognized as a parasite primarily of domestic and farm animals, particularly puppies, kittens, chickens, calves, and sheep.[16] Then, all of a sudden, a cluster of cases were spotted in humans, including an on-going epidemic in Haiti. Dr. Kean asked himself, why was this previously rare, mostly benign disease causing so much havoc in the bowels of his patient and in scores of others in the Caribbean? The patient died in 1983 of unstoppable cryptosporidiosis, and hundreds of additional cases of the disease in its killing form were suddenly being reported in New York and San Francisco.

The occurrences of Kaposi's sarcoma, *P. carinii*, and/or other opportunistic infections in a person with unexplained immune dysfunction soon became known as the *acquired immune deficiency syndrome*, or more simply, AIDS. By early 1982, the disease was known by a variety of names and acronyms. The most popular of these was GRID, for Gay-Related Immune Deficiency. As *The New York Times* reported:

> The cause of the disorder is unknown. Researchers call it A.I.D., for acquired immunodeficiency disease, or GRID, for gay-related immunodeficiency.[17]

The *Times* and others also called it "GRID Syndrome,"[18] but staff members at the Centers for Disease Control despised the acronym and refused to use it, particularly since they were well aware that the disease was not restricted to homosexuals.* Journalist Randy Shilts recalled how the situation appeared in April 1982:

> By now a dizzying array of acronyms was being bandied about as possible monikers for an epidemic that, though ten months old, remained unnamed. Besides GRID, some doctors liked ACIDS, for Acquired Community Immune Deficiency Syndrome, and then others favored CAIDS, for Community Acquired Immune Deficiency Syndrome. The CDC hated GRID and preferred calling it "the epidemic of immune deficiency." The "community" in other versions, of course, was a polite way of saying gay; the doctors couldn't let go of the notion that one identified this disease by whom it hit rather than what it did.[19]

When someone finally suggested the sexually neutral yet snappy acronym "AIDS" during the middle of 1982, it immediately replaced all others.[20]

With the recognition that the vast majority of the early cases of this new clinical syndrome involved homosexual men, it seemed logical that the causes might be related to the lifestyle unique to that population. The so-called "sexual revolution" of the 1960s and 1970s was accompanied not only by a greater level of permissiveness among both heterosexuals and gays, but also by a more positive social acceptance of homosexuality in many communities. The emergence of commercial bathhouses** and other outlets for sexual contacts among gays further increased the opportunities for sexual encounters, with some groups within the male gay population viewing promiscuity as a facet of gay liberation. In fact, among many early patients diagnosed with AIDS, much of the sexual activity with multiple partners typically occurred within the anonymity of the bathhouses. Some had had as many as 20,000 sexual contacts and more than 1,100 sex partners.

Active homosexual men with multiple sex partners were also manifesting high rates of sexually transmitted diseases—gonorrhea, syphilis, genital herpes, anal warts, and hepatitis B.[21] Many also acquired "enteric" diseases, described by Randy Shilts as follows:

> Another problem was enteric diseases, like amebiasis and giardiasis, caused by organisms that lodged themselves in the intestinal tracts of gay men with alarming frequency. At the New York Gay Men's Health Project . . . 30 percent of the patients suffered from gastrointestinal parasites. In San Francisco, incidence of the "Gay Bowel Syndrome," as it was called in medical journals, had increased by 8,000 percent since 1973. Infection with these parasites was a likely effect of anal intercourse, which was apt to put a man in contact with his partner's fecal

---

*Interestingly, however, in 1981, correspondents at the prestigious Lancet proposed calling the disease "gay compromise syndrome." See R. O. Brennan and D. T. Durack, "Gay Compromise Syndrome," Lancet, 2 (1981), pp. 1338-1339.

** Gay bathhouses are examined at length in Chapter Three.

matter, and was virtually a certainty through the then-popular practice of rimming, which the medical journals politely called oral-anal intercourse.[22]

It should not be surprising that such factors as frequent exposure to semen, rectal exposure to semen, the body's exposure to amyl nitrite and butyl nitrite (better known as "poppers," that were used to enhance sexual pleasure and performance), and/or a high frequency of sexually transmitted diseases were themselves considered potential causes of AIDS. At the close of 1981, Time magazine reported on the use of poppers:

> The missing link could be "poppers," drugs like amyl nitrite and butyl nitrite, which are said to enhance orgasm. More than 85 percent of the CDC patients admitted to inhaling them. Another possible explanation is the so-called immunologic theory, says San Francisco's Dr. Robert Bolan. Homosexuals with many sexual partners often contract numerous venereal diseases, intestinal disruptions, mononucleosis, and other infections, explains Bolan. "This constant, chronic stimulation to their immune system may eventually cause the system to collapse."[23]

Yet while it was apparent that AIDS was a new disease, most of the gay lifestyle factors were not particularly new. It was thus difficult immediately to single out specific behaviors that might be related to the emerging epidemic. Nevertheless, in the minds of much of America AIDS was an immunity disease linked to homosexual practices and the homosexual condition. As the spread of AIDS became linked in the public imagination to the very presence of homosexuals, the gay visibility and affirmation of the past decade allowed for some very nasty scapegoating. AIDS had come along just when the old religious, moral, and cultural arguments against homosexuality seemed to be moderating. Some were even asking, "Could it be that Anita Bryant had been right after all?"

For those too young to remember, Anita Bryant had been a beauty queen, a Miss America contender, and a pop singer. In the 1970s, she divided much of her time between being the national spokesperson for the Florida citrus industry and doing concert tours in the state fair and convention circuits. She was also a devout born-again Christian and was assertedly anti-gay. On January 18, 1977—despite highly publicized opposition by Bryant—Miami, Florida, became the first southern city in the United States to pass a gay-rights ordinance, prohibiting housing and employment discrimination against gay men and lesbians.[24] Bryant quickly countered by organizing "Save Our Children," a movement to overthrow the new legislation. In speaking against the ordinance, she announced:

> The ordinance condones immorality and discriminates against my children's rights to grow up in a healthy decent community. Before I yield

to this insidious attack on God and His laws, I will lead such a crusade to stop it as this country has never seen before. If homosexuality were the normal way, God would have made Adam and Bruce.[25]

On March 20th, Bryant took out a full-page ad in the Miami Herald in which she proclaimed:

Homosexuality is nothing new. Cultures throughout history have dealt with homosexuals almost universally with disdain, abhorrence, disgust—even death. The recruitment of our children is absolutely necessary for the survival and growth of homosexuality. Since homosexuals cannot reproduce, they must recruit, must freshen their ranks. And who better qualifies as a likely recruit than a teenage boy or girl who is surging with sexual awareness.[26]

The reactions to Anita Bryant's diatribe were mixed. On one side of the issue, the Arkansas State House of Representatives unanimously passed a special resolution applauding Bryant for her anti-gay crusade. In fact, the lawmaker who introduced the resolution remarked, "When you go against God's law, you have no human rights." Shortly thereafter, in a countywide referendum, voters in Miami repealed the controversial gay rights ordinance by a margin of 2 to 1. In reaction, there was a boycott of Florida orange juice throughout the gay community nationwide; and syndicated columnist Mike Royko named Anita Bryant to his list of "The Ten Most Obnoxious Americans" and questioned:

If God hates gays so much, how come he picked Michelangelo, a known homosexual, to paint the Sistine Chapel while assigning Anita to go on TV and push orange juice?[27]

But in the early 1980s, the notion that AIDS was some form of "gay plague" was quickly extinguished. The disease was suddenly being reported in other populations, such as intravenous and other injection drug users, blood transfusion patients, and hemophiliacs.[28] What these reports suggested to the scientific community was that an infectious etiology for AIDS had to be considered.

EXPLORING THE VIRAL FRONTIER

Almost immediately after the first cases of AIDS were reported in 1981, researchers at the Centers for Disease Control began tracking the disease backward in time to discover its origins. They ultimately determined that the first cases of AIDS in the United States probably occurred in 1977. By early 1982, AIDS had been reported in 15 states, the District of Columbia, and two foreign countries, but the total number of cases remained extremely low—158 men and one woman. Although more than 90 percent of the men were either gay or bisexual, interviews with all of the patients failed to provide any definite clues about the origin of the disease.

Although it was suspected that AIDS might be transmitted through sexual relations among homosexually active men, the first strong evidence for the idea did not emerge until the completion of a case control study in June 1982 by epidemiologists at the Centers for Disease Control.[29] In that investigation, data were obtained on the sexual partners of 13 of the first 19 cases of AIDS among homosexual men in the Los Angeles area. Within five years before the onset of their symptoms, nine had had sexual contact with people who later developed Kaposi's sarcoma or *P. carinii* pneumonia. The nine were also linked to another interconnected series of 40 AIDS cases in 10 different cities by one individual who had developed a number of the manifestations of AIDS and who was later diagnosed with Kaposi's sarcoma. Overall, the investigation of these 40 cases indicated that 20 percent of the initial AIDS cases in the United States were linked through sexual contact—a statistical clustering that was extremely unlikely to have occurred by chance.*

Yet even in the face of this evidence, some still doubted that AIDS was caused by a transmissible agent. However, when AIDS cases began to emerge in other populations—among individuals who had been injected with blood or blood products, but had no other expected risk factors—the transmission vectors for the disease became somewhat clearer. Such cases were confirmed first among people with hemophilia, followed by blood transfusion recipients, and intravenous drug users who shared hypodermic needles. Then, when there were documented cases of AIDS among the heterosexual partners of male injection drug users, it became increasingly evident that AIDS was a sexually transmitted disease, and that "sexual orientation" was not the element that placed people at risk.[30]

In 1983 and 1984, scientists at the Institute Pasteur in Paris and the National Institutes of Health in the United States identified and isolated the cause of AIDS—Human T-Cell Lymphotropic Virus, Type III (HTLV-III), as it was called in the United States, or Lymphadenophy-Associated Virus (LAV), as it was known by French scientists. Later,

---

*Almost a decade after the release of the report on this investigation, Larry Kramer, the well-known gay author and playwright, recalled:

A few friends had died mysteriously. Several others were sick with unrecognized symptoms. An old friend, Dr. Lawrence Maas, was writing in the Native (a gay newspaper) of puzzling appearances of rare cancers and pneumonias in the gay community. And then, on July 3rd, 1981, The New York Times ran, buried on an inside page, its first (and for a tragically long 19 months only one of seven) article, "Rare Cancer Seen in 41 Homosexuals." I don't know why, but I was scared. I'd had many of the sexually transmitted diseases that the article said I shared with these 41 homosexuals.

See Larry Kramer, *Reports from the Holocaust: The Making of an AIDS Activist* (New York: St. Martin's Press, 1989), p. 9.

this virus was renamed human immunodeficiency virus, more commonly known as HIV.*

Specifically, HIV is a retrovirus, a type of infectious agent that had previously been identified as causing many animal diseases. Subsequent studies demonstrated that HIV is transmitted when virus particles or infected cells gain direct access to the bloodstream. This can occur through all forms of sexual intercourse, through the sharing of contaminated injection equipment, blood, and blood products, and through the passing of the virus from infected mothers to their unborn or newborn children. HIV has been isolated from blood, semen, vaginal secretions, urine, cerebrospinal fluid, saliva, tears, and breast milk of infected individuals. Transmission could theoretically occur from contact with any of these fluids, but the concentration of HIV found in saliva and tears is extremely low. Moreover, no cases of HIV infection have been traced to saliva or tears. Within this context, HIV is a continuum of conditions associated with immune dysfunction, and AIDS is best described as a severe manifestation of infection with HIV.

Subsequent to the discovery of HIV, an early priority was to verify fully its association with the diseases in question. Using a variety of different laboratory tests, researchers in virology and molecular biology searched for antibodies against HIV in the blood of AIDS patients. Ultimately, they found that almost 100 percent of AIDS patients had HIV antibodies.[31] The presence of specific antibodies in the blood indicates that a previous infection registered on the body's immune system. The antibody molecules that remain in the bloodstream act as scouts, so to speak; if the virus appears again, the scouts recognize it immediately and attempt to prevent it from getting a foothold.

This research led, in 1985, to the widespread availability of a commercial test for antibodies to HIV. The basic test is an enzyme-linked immunosorbent assay (ELISA). More commonly known as ELISA or EIA, it is not a test for AIDS, nor does it even detect the presence of the virus itself. What the test does indicate is whether HIV has been noticed by an individual's immune system.

IN SEARCH OF PATIENT ZERO

When epidemiologists at the Centers for Disease Control diagrammed the clustering of AIDS patients in their case control study, at

---

*There is more than one strain of human immunodeficiency virus (HIV). HIV-1 is the most common form. A second variety, discovered in late 1985 and subsequently termed human immunodeficiency virus type 2 (HIV-2), was isolated from two West African patients with AIDS. In evolutionary terms, HIV-2 is clearly related to HIV-1. The two viruses are similar in their overall structure and both can cause AIDS. Although differences in the relative infectiousness of HIV-1 and HIV-2 have not yet been fully determined, it would appear that HIV-2 is a less virulent pathogen. For the sake of simplicity, all references to HIV-1 throughout this book are designated as HIV.

its center was an individual they referred to as "Patient Zero," the public health equivalent of "ground zero" (the point at which a nuclear bomb detonates).[32] "Patient Zero" was Gaetan Dugas, a 28-year-old Air Canada flight attendant who was an active homosexual. Either directly, or indirectly through intermediate contacts, Dugas was presumed to have infected at least 40 of the 248 American patients diagnosed with AIDS before April 1982. He was found to have been a sex partner of nine of the first Los Angeles cases, 22 of the New York patients, and nine cases in Miami, Chicago, and several other cities.

As a flight attendant, Dugas could fly free when on vacation. He liked to travel, he was handsome, and he had encountered 250 sexual partners a year over the prior 10 years. As Randy Shilts described him:

> Gaetan was the man everyone wanted. His hair fell boyishly over his forehead. His mouth easily curled into an inviting smile, and his laugh could flood color into a room of black and white. He bought his clothes in the trendiest shops of Paris and London. He vacationed in Mexico and on the Caribbean beaches. Americans tumbled for his soft Quebecois accent and his sensual magnetism . . .[33]

Afflicted with Kaposi's sarcoma in mid-1980, identified in November 1982 as a carrier of what was still being referred to as "gay cancer," and warned of the risk he could pose to his sex partners, Dugas refused to change his lifestyle. Until his death in 1984, he continued to be sexually active, taking no precautions. Oftentimes he would inform his partners, but only after they had had sex. In the gay baths, for example, after being the active participant in anal intercourse, he was known to turn up the lights, point to the purple blotches on his face, and announce, "I've got gay cancer, I'm going to die and so are you."[34]

Although Gaetan Dugas was one of the earliest of the AIDS cases, having been initially infected in the late 1970s, it is unlikely that he was the first. Some of his sexual partners had manifested symptoms of AIDS before he did.* Because of this and other indications, investigators were also looking elsewhere, including Haiti.

As mentioned earlier in this chapter, in mid-1982 cases of severe illness were discovered among young Haitian refugees at Miami's Jackson Memorial Hospital. Several patients died, and at first they were thought to have had severe tuberculosis. Alert pathologists, however, realized that brain toxoplasmosis was the cause of death. Then, strong similarities began showing up in disease manifestations apparent in the Haitians, gay men, and intravenous drug users—a spectrum that

---

*It should be emphasized here that CDC's and Randy Shilts' characterization of Gaetan Dugas and the identification of the epidemic with but one man has been criticized by many observers as both sensationalist and reprehensible. Without question, Dugas was not the first person to have AIDS. Similarly, there is no proof even that he was the source of the infection among the men whom he was purported to have infected.

would become known as "opportunistic infections." Kaposi's sarcoma was evident in a number of Haitians, and their immune systems were found to be indistinguishable from those in other affected groups. However, they denied being intravenous drug users or homosexuals, and when mounting numbers of Haitians in Miami, New York, and elsewhere were reported as afflicted with the new mysterious disease, epidemiologists began seriously to consider the possibility of a "Haitian connection." In this regard, in one of the first books ever written on AIDS, New York immunologist Frederick P. Siegal and cancer researcher Marta Siegal offered the following:

> The demographics of AIDS among Haitians differs somewhat from that of the other groups. The disease was seen initially among recent refugees, the "boat people," mostly black, poor, and male. Some had evidently brought it with them from Haiti, disembarking, already with fevers and sweats, from the small craft that deposited them on American shores. But others who turned up with identical problems had been in the United States for some time, as many as 8–10 years, and, unlike their compatriots, some were middle-class members of the New York community. What did these people have in common, aside from their country of origin?[35]

Other indications led to a focus on Haitians. In September 1978, a 31-year-old French geologist, Claude Chardon, was involved in a serious road accident in Haiti. At the Port-au-Prince Hospital, his left arm had to be amputated. His transfusions were of fresh blood donated by eight Haitian volunteers. In late 1981, well after he had returned to Paris, Chardon began to experience chronic diarrhea and vomiting, as well as rapid weight loss. By April 1982 he was manifesting all of the clinical signs of acquired immune deficiency, and he died several months later of intestinal cryptosporidiosis and cerebral toxoplasmosis.[36] Another French scientist, this one 40 years old, had moved from France to Haiti in 1978 to live with a young island woman. Four years later he returned to France and fell ill, dying of cerebral toxoplasmosis.[37] There were other cases, and as the Yugoslav-Parisian physician Mirko Grmek reflected years later:

> American epidemiologists, in an exquisite twist of black humor, called the most exposed groups the "Four-H Club": homosexuals, Haitians, heroin addicts, and hemophiliacs. Some replaced the last group with hookers, bringing in fact the fateful club membership to five. To reassure the public, two "innocent" groups were omitted from this club of the damned: recipients of blood transfusions and newborns infected in utero.[38]

In retrospect, the classification of Haitians as an AIDS "risk group" was unwarranted, for there was never any evidence to support such a conjectural theory. Or as Paul Farmer of Harvard Medical School commented:

> The Haitian cases and subsequent "risk-grouping" spurred the publication of a wide range of theories purporting to explain the epidemiology and origins of AIDS. In December 1982, for example, a physician with the U.S. National Cancer Institute was widely quoted as announcing that "we suspect that this may be an epidemic Haitian virus that was brought back to the homosexual population in the United States."[39]

This theory, however, was unbolstered by research and served only to blame and scapegoat an entire culture. In retrospect, Dr. Farmer's analysis of AIDS in Haiti is an important one. As a physician and anthropologist, he conducted research in Haiti for almost a decade. Drawing on his own work and more recent epidemiological research, he demonstrated that AIDS developed in Haiti in much the same way that it emerged in the United States, hitting male gay communities and recipients of blood transfusions. Only later, as Haiti sunk into economic despair and scores of both men and women become involved in prostitution as a means of economic support, did AIDS enter the heterosexual population.

AIDS AND AFRICA

Where did AIDS and HIV actually originate? The matter remains unsettled. However, considerable attention has been given to Central Africa. The AIDS problem in Africa first became evident in 1982 when physicians in Belgium began seeing patients from Zaire and Burundi.[40] Prior to gaining their independence in the early 1960s, Zaire and Burundi had been part of the Belgian Congo, and for many years citizens with financial means still traveled to Belgium for their major medical care. Some patients had signs and symptoms virtually identical to what was being called AIDS in the United States. Investigation led to a number of different theories. The first was that HIV had existed for decades, nestled in remote regions of Africa and limited to small, relatively isolated populations.[41] The social mores and behavior of those populations may not have been conducive to the rapid spread of the disease, and the few cases that did develop could likely have escaped detection against the backdrop of multiple life-threatening infections that are common to the region.

There were a number of factors that eventually changed this pattern. African cities grew dramatically after World War II, principally the result of independence. As in other parts of the world, the urbanization of Africa was accompanied by social changes and family disruptions, combined with the anonymity of urban life—all of which increased the likelihood of behaviors that contributed to the spread of sexually transmitted diseases. Multiple sex partners and prostitution were among the signs of these changes. In time, the prevalence of HIV increased sufficiently to make AIDS visible as a new clinical entity in Africa and elsewhere.

An alternative theory suggests that the natural home of the AIDS virus is in an animal. The African green monkey was singled out as one of the prime suspects. This hypothesis suggested that somehow the virus mutated and jumped species, entering the human population when monkeys bit hunters who were attempting to capture them for food.[42]

Several investigations have also suggested that AIDS and HIV may have made their way to North America from Africa, via Haiti. More specifically, from the early 1960s through the mid-1970s, there was considerable migration from Zaire to Haiti, and many of these immigrants are believed to have settled in the United States.[43] In addition, several of the early commentators on the epidemic argued that African green monkeys were imported to Haiti from Zaire and kept as pets in male houses of prostitution.[44] And finally, there was the point of view that Haiti was a popular vacation spot for gay Americans, who brought the disease home with them and infected the mainland population.[45] But again, the theories linking AIDS to Haiti should not be accepted uncritically, for evidence of such a link continues to be lacking.

Whatever the source or sources, by 1983 it was clear that AIDS was an epidemic disease with a virtual 100 percent mortality rate. But what was most puzzling to a few virologists and epidemiologists was their feelings of *déjà vu* when reviewing some of their earlier case notes and other reports in the literature. Although medical epidemiologic research and conventional wisdom date the beginnings of the epidemic in Africa, Europe, Haiti, and the United States to the late 1970s, there was evidence that the disease appeared earlier in several locales, thus contributing further to the overall medical mystery.

Several retrospective reports of cases resembling AIDS both clinically and immunologically appeared in the literature in the years following the discovery of HIV.[46] Typically, however, conclusive evidence of HIV infection in these cases had not been (or could not be) documented. But in other cases the evidence was more convincing. A previously healthy, 32-year-old, heterosexual Canadian man who received a blood transfusion in Zaire in 1976 represents an interesting example.[47] Twelve days after his plane had crashed in a remote section of Zaire, he was found by a group of villagers and was transported to Kisingani University. As he had suffered a compound fracture in his right leg, his treatment included a blood transfusion. After his transfer to a hospital in Canada, he began to manifest symptoms of a variety of opportunistic infections. He died in June 1980, and postmortem examination revealed findings similar to those described in cases of AIDS.[48] Serologic testing in 1983 of stored blood drawn several months before his death repeatedly had positive results for HIV antibodies. When the physician who treated this patient in Zaire was contacted, he reported that local villagers had come to the hospital to donate blood for his transfusion, suggesting that transfusion-related AIDS cases dated to the mid-1970s, and that HIV was present in Zaire prior to the known beginnings of the epidemic.

An even earlier case involved a Norwegian child and her parents.[49] The father, born in 1946, exhibited clinical and immunological manifestations of AIDS beginning in 1966; the mother, born in 1943, had similar manifestations starting in 1967; and the child, born in 1967, became ill with bacterial and other recurring infections at two years of age. All three members of the family died in 1976, and subsequent assays of stored blood samples were found to be HIV positive. The child would appear to be the first recorded case of pediatric AIDS, and the family members as a whole represent the first proven case of AIDS in Europe. The case history of the father suggests that he may have contracted the infection in Africa. He was a sailor who had visited a number of African ports, several times prior to 1966. He had contracted sexually transmitted diseases on at least two occasions during his travels, and no other known risk factors for HIV were present in his family.

The first AIDS case in the United States may also date back to the 1960s. It involved a 15-year-old boy who had been admitted to St. Louis City Hospital suffering from extensive swelling of his legs, penis, and scrotum.[50] He had no history of intravenous drug use, blood transfusions, or travel outside the Midwest. He did admit to being sexually active, engaging in anal intercourse, and it was suspected that he may have been gay. In addition to the swelling, he was suffering from a number of infections, and he continued to deteriorate. He died 16 months later. The postmortem examination revealed that he had Kaposi's sarcoma—at that time an extremely rare cancer in the United States. Because the physicians at the St. Louis hospital were at a loss to explain the cause and course of the youth's condition, blood and tissue samples were frozen for later analysis. Subsequent study of the samples found a retrovirus related to HIV.

These cases suggest that HIV or a genetically related virus may have entered several communities before the current epidemic began. In each case, however, the virus failed to gain a foothold in a large, sexually active or drug/needle-sharing population. When each lone carrier died, the potential chain of infection was broken.

THE AIDS CONSPIRACIES

In a lecture delivered at Oxford University in November 1963, the late and eminent Pulitzer Prize-winning American historian, Richard Hofstadter, offered some reflections on what he called a "paranoid style" in American politics.[51] He was referring to the qualities of heated exaggeration, suspiciousness, and conspiratorial fantasy regarding certain social issues that were often characteristic of a small minority of "angry minds" in the American political establishment. But he distinguished his concept from that of clinical paranoia:

> Webster defines paranoia, the clinical entity, as a chronic mental disorder characterized by systematized delusions of persecution and of one's own greatness. In the paranoid style, as I conceive it, the feeling of persecution is central, and it is indeed systematized in grandiose theories of conspiracy.[52]

Professor Hofstadter went on to consider further vital differences between the paranoid in politics and the clinical paranoiac:

> . . . although they both tend to be overheated, oversuspicious, overaggressive, grandiose, and apocalyptic in expression, the clinical paranoid sees the hostile and conspiratorial world in which he feels himself living as directed specifically against him; whereas the spokesman of the paranoid style finds it directed against a nation, a culture, a way of life whose fate affects not only himself but millions of others.[53]

One can readily call up numerous examples of the paranoid style in American political history, remembering that Hofstadter's thoughts had come just after 20 years of post-World War II anxiety about treason and conspiracy in the United States. The view that President Franklin D. Roosevelt had sold out Eastern Europe to Stalin at the Yalta Conference in 1945 was an early expression of this paranoia, fostering the notion that there was a sinister conspiracy to destroy America from within. Then, in March 1947, President Harry S. Truman inadvertently fueled anxieties by ordering all government employees to sign "loyalty oaths"—statements that they did not belong to the Communist Party or to other groups suspected of disloyalty. During the 1950s, there was the arrest, conviction, and execution of Julius and Ethel Rosenberg for giving atomic secrets to the Soviet Union, as well as Senator Joseph McCarthy's ravings about "communists in our midst." In the same vein were the conspiratorial explanations of President John F. Kennedy's assassination, most recently revisited in Oliver Stone's $40 million motion picture conspiracy epic, JFK, in 1991.*

---

*In all likelihood, it would appear that the J.F.K. conspiracy theory may never die. In June 1993, when former Texas Governor John Connally died of natural causes, requests were made of his family that his body be exhumed in a new search for evidence about John F. Kennedy's assassination. Connally had been wounded when riding in the motorcade with

In reflecting upon the paranoid style, quite clearly the fashion is not necessarily limited to members of the political community. Consider, for example, how the Ku Klux Klan and other neo-Nazi hate groups view minority group integration as a threat to the existence of the white race,[54] or how the National Rifle Association sees any form of gun control as movement toward the apocalyptic worlds of Mad Max and The Road Warrior. Characteristic of these varieties of the paranoid style are leaps into fantasy, fear mongering, and hopeless pessimism, with the perceived enemies characterized as amoral and sinister.

In retrospect, there is much in the history and rhetoric of the AIDS crisis that reflects the paranoid style, for conspiracy theories as to the origins of AIDS have been abundant. Among the first to surface were those suggesting that the virus had been developed specifically to target gay men. For example, in a leaflet distributed in 1983 by the Communistcadre, a self-styled scientific Trotskyist group, it was proclaimed that "AIDS is political germ warfare by the U.S. government . . . to generate a serious epidemic among gay men."[55] Similar theories appeared from time to time in the gay press, including one suggesting that a chemical agent had been "sprinkled like fairy dust on the floors of bathhouses where barefoot homosexuals would absorb it through their skin."[56]

A widely circulated opinion as to the origin of AIDS was published in numerous Soviet outlets. During the summer months of 1987, several Soviet-sponsored articles stated that the AIDS virus had been created by Pentagon experiments; that the research had been carried out at Fort Detrick, Maryland; and that it was initiated to develop a subtle biological weapon. The articles appeared not only in Soviet outlets, but in newspapers in Kenya, Peru, Sudan, Nigeria, Mexico, and Senegal as well. On November 4, 1987, however, members of the Soviet Academy of Sciences distanced themselves from the rumor, and their disavowals were published in Izvestia, the Soviet government newspaper.[57]

Among the more preposterous and undocumented theories of AIDS was one that was asserted in 1988 by Los Angeles dermatologist Alan Cantwell.[58] As in the Soviet press report, Cantwell announced that AIDS was the result of a man-made, genetically-engineered virus that was either deliberately or accidently introduced into selected populations as part of a secret scientific germ-warfare experiment. More specifically, he contended that the outbreaks of AIDS in New York City, San

---

President Kennedy when he was shot. Researchers suggested that bullet fragments, which may have remained in Connally's body, could show whether a second gun, and hence a second marksman, was involved in the shooting (see *The New York Times*, 19 June 1993, p. 6). And if this wasn't enough, at about the same time, a documentary on National Public Radio, The RFK Tapes, proposed that the assassination of Robert F. Kennedy in 1968 had also been a conspiracy, and that Sirhan Sirhan, the convicted assassin, had been a brainwashed setup for the real killer (see *Time*, 7 June 1993, p. 45).

Francisco, and Los Angeles at the close of the 1970s were the result of government-sponsored viral vaccine research that used gay men as human guinea pigs. He also argued that AIDS may have been introduced into Central Africa by vaccine programs sponsored by the World Health Organization. His final point was that a massive cover-up by the combined forces of the government and the nation's scientific community managed to keep this information from the American public.

In a letter dated February 25, 1987, written and widely circulated by Frances Cress Welsing, a Washington, D.C., psychiatrist, an alternative theory of AIDS as a "man-made" virus was forcefully presented. Reminding readers of the Tuskegee syphilis experiments,* Dr. Welsing implied that AIDS was an instrument of genocide, likely introduced into black and other "undesirable" populations for the purpose of a systematic depopulation agenda.[59] To support her contention, Dr. Welsing quoted the following paragraph from the 1969 treatise *A Survey of Chemical and Biological Warfare*:

> The question of whether new diseases could be used [for biological warfare] is of considerable interest. Vervet monkey disease may well be an example of a whole new class of disease-causing organisms. Handling of blood and tissues without precautions causes infection. It is unaffected by any antibiotic substance so far tried and is unrelated to any other organism. It causes fatality in some cases and can be venereally transmitted in man.[60]

Dr. Welsing pointed out that the vervet monkey was none other than the African green monkey—already implicated in other hypotheses about the origins of AIDS.

Dr. Welsing's theory is easily refuted, for the disease of which she spoke is of a category known as *viral hemorrhagic fever*. In 1967, an outbreak of a particular strain of hemorrhagic fever occurred in Germany and Yugoslavia among laboratory workers engaged in processing kidneys from African green monkeys for cell culture production. The disease also attacked the medical personnel attending the initial group

---

*The Tuskegee Study, as it has come to be known, involved a sample of some 400 syphilitic black men in Macon County, Alabama, who were deliberately denied treatment. The purpose of the study was to determine the course and complications of untreated, latent syphilis in black males and to ascertain whether it differed from the course of the disease in whites. Syphilitic men chosen for the Tuskegee sample were told that they were ill and were promised free care. Unaware that they were participants in an experiment, all subjects believed that they were being treated for "bad blood"—a rural South colloquialism for syphilis. The project endured from 1932 through 1972, undertaken with the complicity of the United States Public Health Service. For the full story of the Tuskegee Study, see Molly Selvin, "Changing Medical and Social Attitudes Toward Sexually Transmitted Diseases: A Historical Overview," in King K. Holmes, Per-Anders Mardh, P. Frederick Sparling, and Paul J. Wiesner, eds., *Sexually Transmitted Diseases* (New York: McGraw-Hill,1984), pp. 13-14; J.H. Jones, *Bad Blood: The Scandalous Story of the Tuskegee Experiment* (New York: Free Press, 1981).

of patients. There were a total of 31 cases, of which several were fatal. A virus was isolated from the blood and tissues of the patients. Named Marburg virus after the town in Germany where the first cases were described, it was found to be unique and unrelated to any other known human pathogen.[61]

In subsequent years there were a few small and short-lived outbreaks of the disease, and clinical studies found that the spread had occurred through close contact with infected persons, or through contact with infected blood or body secretions or excretions.[62] Sexual transmission of the disease has occurred, and the virus has been isolated from seminal fluid up to two months after illness.[63] Although this might suggest some similarities with HIV infection, the incubation period for Marburg virus ranges from only three to nine days—a marked difference with the months to years between initial HIV infection and the appearance of AIDS.

Although speculative and conspiratorial theories of AIDS attract little attention and tend to fade as quickly as they appear, there was one exception. A relatively new hypothesis was published in the March 19, 1992, issue of *Rolling Stone*,[64] and it quickly drew the attention of scientists throughout the nation. The author of the article, Houston free-lance writer Tom Curtis, speculated that some as-yet-undiscovered *simian* (monkey) form of HIV may have contaminated a polio vaccine formulated decades ago by researchers at the prestigious Wistar Institute in Philadelphia. Curtis suggested that the antecedent virus might have come from monkey kidney cells in which the polio vaccine had been cultured. The vaccine had been tested during the late 1950s in what is now Zaire, Rwanda, and Burundi, where it was spray-injected into the mouths of several hundred thousand people. Piling speculation upon speculation, Curtis intimated that HIV infection might have occurred through mucosal cells, lesions in the mouth, or via aerosolized virus trickling into the lungs.

To those unfamiliar with the nature of viruses and the production of vaccines, the *Rolling Stone* thesis seemed plausible. In the first place, the Wistar Institute had indeed used monkeys in the preparation of the polio vaccine. Secondly, the vaccine was widely distributed in the Belgian Congo in the late 1950s. Perhaps most importantly, there are numerous HIV-related viruses found in monkeys.[65] Soon after the recognition of AIDS in people, several clinical reports described outbreaks of severe infections, wasting disease,* and death in several colonies of

---

*"Wasting" disease is a characterized by involuntary weight loss combined with chronic diarrhea, fever, fatigue, and weakness. In parts of Central Africa, this illness in humans is often referred to as "slim" disease.

During late 1982, a new epidemic disease was reported in a small village on the shores of Lake Victoria near the Uganda-Tanzania border. Seventeen people were complaining of intestinal troubles and weight loss. Since all of the patients were smugglers, it became known as the "robbers" disease. But when the illness began attacking others whose

Asian macaque monkeys housed at primate centers in the United States.[66] This was subsequently referred to as simian AIDS (or SAIDS), and SIV (simian immunodeficiency virus) was found to be the causative agent. The SIVs constitute a family of naturally occurring viruses indigenous to certain simian species in Africa. In their natural hosts—African green monkeys, sooty mangabeys, and mandrills—they apparently cause no disease. But accidental infection of macaques with certain strains of SIV causes persistent infection, with eventual death from simian AIDS.[67]

By contrast, there was no real evidence to support the Curtis thesis that appeared in *Rolling Stone*. When his work was severely criticized by AIDS researchers for its lack of documentation, Curtis admitted that, unlike science, journalism allows for theories without hard proof.[68]

The purported conspiracies surrounding the origins of AIDS, the assassinations of John and Robert Kennedy, and the benign forms of paranoia that result in Elvis and Hitler spottings—all in the face of little or no supporting evidence—are difficult to understand. Perhaps they reflect a need to decipher life's baffling and inexplicable dark sides, or a sense of impotency in the face of events that cannot be controlled. With respect to AIDS, they may be an outgrowth of many Americans' spirit of individualism, which encourages an instinctive distrust of authority and officialdom. Or they may be something else. Ken Kesey, author of *One Flew Over the Cuckoo's Nest*, advanced a theory of his own in 1986:

> You know, some people say syphilis came from screwing sheep and pigs, and there are some who say that AIDS may have come from monkeys. So, when the scriptures, not just the Judeo-Christian scriptures, but lots of scriptures say, "Don't screw animals," it's not because God doesn't want us screwing animals, he's telling us that if we're going to screw animals, we're going to get things from them. What we've really not dealt with is what if this is not a virus? What if we're manufacturing it? What if by adding billions and billions of sperm cells to membranes that are not supposed to handle sperm, you begin to come up with something that is different?[69]

---

honesty was not in doubt, it was called "slim." The name came from the English word connoting an extremely lean condition, because in the later stages of the disease the patients resembled living skeletons before they eventually died in a state of total debilitation.

In 1987, slim was included in the Centers for Disease Control's definition of AIDS. See D. Serwadda, R.D. Mugerwa, and N.K. Sewankambo, "Slim Disease: A New Disease in Uganda and its Association with HTLV-III/LAV Infection," *Lancet*, 2 (1985), pp. 849-852; Centers for Disease Control, "Revision of the CDC Surveillance Case Definition for Acquired Immunodeficiency Syndrome," *Morbidity and Mortality Weekly Report*, 36, Suppl (1987), pp. 3-15.

POSTSCRIPT

Because the majority of AIDS cases were concentrated in what were considered to be "deviant" groups in the United States—gays and intravenous drug users—during the first few years after the discovery of the virus, AIDS seemed to be an invisible epidemic. On July 21, 1983, for example, while virologists and medical epidemiologists throughout the world were struggling to understand this new, unusual, and very clever virus of uncertain origins, the notable historian William McNeill made the following comment in the *New York Review of Books*:

> One of the things that separates us from our ancestors and makes contemporary experience profoundly different from that of other ages is the disappearance of epidemic disease as a serious factor in human life. Nowadays if a few score of people die of an infection, officials declare an epidemic, the newspapers are full of it, and medical resources are quickly marshalled to find the source and check the further progress of the disease.[70]

These were the opening words of McNeill's review of Robert S. Gottfried's *The Black Death*,[71] the newest history and analysis of that mid-fourteenth century plague that seems to epitomize the catastrophe of epidemic disease in the minds of most people. Curiously, in McNeill's 3000-word essay, written by a person well versed in the dynamics of plagues and at a time when stories of AIDS had begun to appear in the press, the newly emergent disease was completely ignored. The major television networks also side-stepped the new affliction. NBC's Robert Bazell was the first reporter to broadcast an AIDS story on the influential evening news, on June 17, 1982. This was decidedly a late start by the TV giant, but it was earlier than ABC by four months, and a good year and a half before anything was heard from CBS.[72]

When the princes and talking heads of the evening broadcast journalism fraternity finally got into the business of AIDS reporting, their manner of presentation often served mostly to confuse, obscure, garble, and misrepresent the message. One of the better examples in this regard was David Brinkley on the June 18, 1983, broadcast of ABC's "World News Tonight." His news item was as follows:

> The terrible new disease, AIDS, first seen among homosexuals, drug users, Haitians, and hemophiliacs, is now appearing among people who are none of these. A study in the *New England Journal of Medicine* says apparently the disease can be spread by contact between heterosexuals—and there's no cure in sight.[73]

Brinkley's 20-second feature started telephones ringing around the country to physicians and scientists from alarmed Americans in all fifty states. Technically, what Brinkley had conveyed was correct, however incomplete. The networks and news anchors have never been known for their sexual straight talk, and had Brinkley simply inserted the word "sexual" before the phrase "contact between heterosexuals," much fear, consternation, and confusion could have been avoided. Many asked: "Does this mean that AIDS can spread casually, through a cough or sneeze, by a handshake, grasping a doorknob, or from sitting on a toilet seat?" Dan Rather of CBS did not help matters when he gravely looked into the camera one evening and pronounced that AIDS was being spread by "household contact."[74]

Even after the media had finally discovered the AIDS epidemic, it remained invisible to much of the federal bureaucracy. The Reagan administration, in particular, was remarkably slow to respond. From the very beginning, virologists and epidemiologists at the Centers for Disease Control, the National Cancer Institute, and the National Institute of Allergy and Infectious Diseases were active in tracking and identifying the new virus, and physicians and researchers at the major hospitals in New York, San Francisco, Miami, and Los Angeles began some of the first clinical studies of AIDS in the United States. However, federal funding for AIDS research was minimal.[75]

What finally brought AIDS "out of the closet," so to speak, was actor Rock Hudson. On July 25, 1985, Hudson's AIDS diagnosis was announced. On that day, the plague finally touched America. It was also the first time that President Reagan expressed concern for the sufferings of those dying from AIDS.[76] Reagan's first public uttering of the word AIDS came later that year, on September 17th, when he offered his empathy for parents who did not want their youngsters "in school with kids with AIDS."[77] Reagan's first speech on AIDS did not come until the night of May 31, 1987, almost a decade into the epidemic. Earlier that day, Larry Kramer had written in *New York Newsday*:

> Tonight, the President of all the American people is finally going to make his first AIDS speech.
>
> He will address a fund-raising dinner of the American Foundation for AIDS Research. He will speak on the eve of the Third International Conference on AIDS, which is expected to draw six thousand attendees to Washington, twice last year's attendance in Paris.
>
> He will tell us that AIDS is awful and that it's his administration's No. 1 health priority, hollow assertions that have been voiced by somebody or other in his administration since 1983. He may talk about his new advisory commission on AIDS, about "education," and about testing.
>
> But what will really count is how long and how seriously Ronald Reagan addresses the issues of research and treatment—the launching of an all-out federal war to find a cure for this plague. Even if he mentions these subjects, it is perfectly clear to me that no matter what Reagan

says tonight, it's not going to alter the sorry journal of these plague years.[78]

Reagan's first AIDS speech was received with boos—three rounds of booing in all. He never used the words "gay" or "homosexual," and he made no mention of the long-awaited federal "war" on AIDS. He did announce that he favored mandatory AIDS testing, and he praised heterosexual AIDS service organizations. When George Bush spoke the following day at the opening ceremonies of the AIDS conference, he was booed even louder—by gay activists and non-gays alike.[79]

END NOTES

1. Erik Eckholm, "River Blindness: Conquering an Ancient Scourge," *The New York Times Magazine*, 8 Jan. 1989, pp. 20–27, 58–59.

2. Randy Shilts, *And the Band Played On: Politics, People, and the AIDS Epidemic* (New York: St. Martin's Press, 1987), pp. 3–4, 118.

3. World Health Organization/International Commission to Sudan, 1976, "Ebola Hemorrhagic Fever in Sudan," *Bulletin of the World Health Organization*, 56 (1978), pp. 247–270; World Health Organization/International Commission to Zaire, 1976, "Ebola Hemorrhagic fever in Zaire," *Bulletin of the World Health Organization*, 56 (1978), pp. 271–293.

4. See Geoffrey Eu, *Amazon Wildlife* (Hong Kong: APA Publications, 1992), p. 107; Redmond O'Hanlon, *In Trouble Again: A Journey Between the Orinoco and the Amazon* (New York: Vintage Press, 1990), p. 1.

5. Jonathan Leonard, "Carlos Chagas, Health Pioneer of the Brazilian Backlands," *Bulletin of PAHO*, 24 (1990), pp. 226–239.

6. Achilea L. Bittencourt, Moises Sadigursky, Antusa A. Da Silva, Carlos A. S. Menezes, Mercia M. M. Marianetti, Solon C. Guerra, and Italo Sherlock, "Evaluation of Chagas' Disease Transmission Through Breast–Feeding," *Memorial Institute of Oswaldo Cruz*, 83 (1988), pp. 37–39.

7. Bittencourt et al.

8. Centers for Disease Control, "Pneumocystis Pneumonia—Los Angeles," *Morbidity and Mortality Weekly Report*, 30 (5 June 1981), pp. 250–252; Centers for Disease Control, "Kaposi's Sarcoma and Pneumocystis Pneumonia Among Homosexual Men—New York City and California," *Morbidity and Mortality Weekly Report*, 30 (3 July 1981), pp. 305–308; M. S. Gottlieb, R. Schroff, H. Schanker, J. D. Weismal, P. T. Fan, R. A. Wolf, and A. Saxon, "Pneumocystis Carinii Pneumonia and Mucosal Candidiasis in Previously Healthy Homosexual Men: Evidence of a New Acquired Cellular Immunodeficiency," New England Journal of Medicine, 305 (10 Dec. 1981), pp. 1425–1431; H. Masur, M. A. Michelis, J. B. Greene, I. Onorato, R. A. Vande Stouwe, R. T. Holzman, G. Wormser, L. Brettmen, M. Lange, H. W. Murray, and S. Cunningham–Rundles, "An Outbreak of Community–Acquired Pneumocystis Carinii Pneumonia: Initial Manifestation of Cellular Immune Dysfunction," *New England Journal of Medicine*, 305 (1981), pp. 1431–1438.

9. *The New York Times*, 5 July 1981, p. E7.

10. Anthony Martinez, Anthony F. Suffredini, and Henry Masur, "*Pneumocystis Carinii* Disease in HIV–Infected Persons," in Gary P. Wormser (ed.), *AIDS and Other Manifestations of HIV Infection* (New York: Raven Press, 1992), pp. 225–247.

11. Jeffrey A. Golden, "Pulmonary Complications of AIDS," in Jay A. Levy (ed.), *AIDS: Pathogenesis and Treatment* (New York: Marcel Dekker, 1989), pp. 403–447; W. T. Hughes, "Pneumocystis Carinii, "in G. L. Mandell, R. G. Douglous, and J. E. Bennett (eds.), *Principles and Practices of Infectious Diseases* (New York: John Wiley, 1979), pp. 2137–2142.

12. See P. A. Volberding, M. A. Conant, R. B. Strickler, and B. J. Lewis, "Chemotherapy in Advanced Kaposi's Sarcoma: Implications for Current Cases in Homosexual Men," *American Journal of Medicine* 74 (1983), pp. 652–

656; Bureau of Hygiene and Tropical Diseases, "Kaposi's Sarcoma: More Questions Than Answers," *WorldAIDS*, Nov. 1990, p. 11.

13. Dennis Altman, *AIDS in the Mind of America: The Social, Political, and Psychological Impact of the New Epidemic* (Garden City, NY: Anchor Books, 1987), pp. 36–37.

14. Joseph A. Kovacs and Henry Masur, "Opportunistic Infections," in Vincent T. DeVita, Samuel Hellman, and Steven A. Rosenberg (eds.), *AIDS: Etiology, Diagnosis, Treatment, and Prevention* (Philadelphia: Lippincott, 1988), pp. 199–225.

15. B. H. Kean, *M.D.* (New York: Ballantine Books, 1990), pp. 391–402.

16. Frederick P. Siegal and Marta Siegal, *AIDS: The Medical Mystery* (New York: Grove Press, 1983), p. 25.

17. *The New York Times*, 11 May 1982, p. C1.

18. *The New York Times*, 18 June 1982, p. B8.

19. Shilts, p. 138.

20. Shilts, p. 171.

21. Anne Rompalo and H. Hunter Handsfield, "Overview of Sexually Transmitted Diseases in Homosexual Men," in Pearl Ma and Donald Armstrong, (eds.), *AIDS and Infections of Homosexual Men* (Boston: Butterworths, 1989), pp. 3–11.

22. Shilts, pp. 18–19.

23. *Time*, 21 Dec. 1981, p. 68.

24. Peter N. Carroll, *It Seemed Like Nothing Happened: The Tragedy and Promise of America in the 1970s* (New York: Holt, Rinehart and Winston, 1982), p. 290.

25. Carroll, pp. 290–291.

26. *Miami Herald*, 20 March 1977.

27. Leigh W. Rutledge, *The Gay Decades* (New York: Plume Books, 1992), pp. 100–112.

28. Centers for Disease Control, "Epidemiologic Aspects of the Current Outbreak of Kaposi's Sarcoma and Opportunistic Infections," *New England Journal of Medicine*, 306 (1982), pp. 248–252.

29. D. M. Auerbach, W. W. Darrow, H. W. Jaffe, and J. W. Curran, "Cluster of Cases of Acquired Immune Deficiency Syndrome: Patients Linked by Sexual Contact," *American Journal of Medicine*, 76 (1984), pp. 487–492.

30. Ann Giudici Fettner, "The Discovery of AIDS: Perspectives from a Medical Journalist," in Gary P. Wormser, Rosalyn E. Stahl, and Edward J. Bottone (eds.), *AIDS and Other Manifestations of HIV Infection* (Park Ridge, NJ: Noyes Publications, 1987), pp. 2–17.

31. Institute of Medicine, National Academy of Sciences, *Mobilizing Against AIDS: The Unfinished Story of a Virus* (Cambridge: Harvard University Press, 1986), p. 20.

32. Robin Marantz Henig, *A Dancing Matrix: Voyages Along the Viral Frontier* (New York: Alfred A. Knopf, 1993), p. 38.

33. Shilts, p. 21.

34. Mirko D. Grmek, *History of AIDS: Emergence and Origin of a Modern Pandemic* (Princeton, NJ: Princeton University Press, 1990), p. 19; Shilts, p. 165.

35. Siegal and Siegal, p. 82.

36. T. Andreani, R. Modigliani, and Y. LeCharpentier, "Acquired Immunodeficiency with Intestinal Cryptoporidiosis: Possible Transmission by Haitian Whole Blood," *Lancet 1* (1983), pp. 1187–1190.

37. Grmek, p. 27.

38. Grmek, p. 31.

39. Paul Farmer, *AIDS and Accusation: Haiti and the Geography of Blame* (Berkeley: University of California Press, 1992), p. 2.

40. N. J. Clumeck, H. Sonnett, and H. Taelman, "Acquired Immunodeficiency Syndrome in African Patients," *New England Journal of Medicine*, 210 (1984), pp. 492–497.

41. Institute of Medicine, National Academy of Sciences, *Mobilizing Against AIDS: The Unfinished Story of a Virus* (Cambridge: Harvard University Press, 1989), p. 107.

42. See Max Essex and Phyllis J. Kanki, "The Origins of the AIDS Virus," in Jonathan Piel, ed. *The Science of AIDS* (New York: W. H. Freeman, 1989), pp. 27–37; *The New York Times*, 21 Nov. 1985, p. A1.

43. Vincent T. DeVita, Samuel Hellman, and Steven A. Rosenberg, *AIDS: Etiology, Diagnosis, Treatment, and Prevention* (Philadelphia: J.B. Lippincott, 1985), p. 304.

44. Dennis Altman, *AIDS in the Mind of America: The Social, Political, and Psychological Impact of the New Epidemic* (Garden City, NY: Doubleday, 1987), p. 72; *Newsweek*, 7 May 1984, pp. 101–102.

45. Altman, p. 72.

46. H. P. Katner and G. A. Pankey "Evidence of a Euro–American Origin of Human Immunodeficiency Virus (HIV)," *Journal of the National Medical Association*, 79 (1987), pp. 1068–1072; D. Huminer and S. D. Pitlik, "Further Evidence for the Existence of AIDS in the Pre–AIDS Era," *Reviews of Infectious Diseases*, 10 (1988), p. 1061.

47. E. Rogan, L. D. Jewell, B. W. Meilke, D. Kunimoto, A. Voth, and D. L. Tyrrell, "A Case of Acquired Immune Deficiency Syndrome Before 1980," *Canadian Medical Association Journal*, 137 (1987), pp. 637–638.

48. C. Reichert, T. Giliary, and D. Levens, "Autopsy Pathology in the Acquired Immune Deficiency Syndrome," *American Journal of Pathology*, 112 (1983), pp. 357–382.

49. S. S. Froland, P. Jenum, C. F. Lindboe, K. W. Wefring, P. J. Linnestad, and T. Bohmer, "HIV–1 Infection in Norwegian Family Before 1970," *Lancet* (11 June 1988), pp. 1344–1345.

50. R. F. Garry, M. H. Witte, A. Gottlieb, M. Elvin–Lewis, M. S. Gottlieb, C. L. Witte, S. S. Alesander, W. R. Cole, and W. L. Drake, "Documentation of an AIDS Virus Infection in the United States in 1968," *Journal of the American Medical Association*, 260 (1988), pp. 2085–2087.

51. Richard Hofstadter, *The Paranoid Style of American Politics and Other Essays* (New York: Alfred A. Knopf, 1965).

52. Hofstadter, p. 4.

53. Hofstadter, p. 4.

54. See *Newsweek*, 29 April 1985, pp. 34–35; *Newsweek*, 4 March 1985, pp. 23–26; *Time*, 18 Feb. 1985, p. 42.

55. Altman, p. 43.

56. Altman, p. 43.

57. See *The New York Times*, 5 Nov. 1987, p. A31.

58. Alan Cantwell, *AIDS and the Doctors of Death: An Inquiry into the Origin of the AIDS Epidemic* (Los Angeles: Aries Rising Press, 1988).

59. Frances Cress Welsing, Unpublished letter, Washington, D.C., 25 Feb. 1987.

60. J. Cookson and J. Nottingham, *A Survey of Chemical and Biological Warfare* (New York: Monthly Review Press, 1969), pp. 322–323.

61. Frederick A. Murphy, "Marburg and Ebola Viruses," in Bernard N. Fields (ed.), *Virology* (New York: Raven Press, 1985), pp. 1111–1118; G. A. Martini and R. Siegert, *Marburg Virus Disease* (Berlin: Springer–Verlag, 1971).

62. J. P. Luby and C. V. Sanders, "Green Monkey Disease ('Marburg Virus' Disease): A New Zoonosis," *Annals of Internal Medicine*, 17 (1969), pp. 657–660; F. W. Van der Walls, K. L. Pomeroy, J. Goudsmit, D. M. Asher, and D. C. Gajdusek, "Hemorrhagic Fever Virus Infections in an Isolated Rainforest Area of Central Liberia: Limitations of the Indirect Immunofluorescence Slide Test for Antibody Screening in Africa," *Tropical and Geographical Medicine*, 38 (1986), pp. 209–214; J. S. S. Gear, G. A. Cassel, A. J. Gear, B. Trappler, L. Clausen, A. M. Meyers, M. C. Kew, T. H. Bothwell, R. Sher, G. B. Miller, J. Schneider, H. J. Koornhof, E. D. Gomperts, M. Isaacson, and J. H. S. Gear, "Outbreak of Marburg Virus Disease in Johannesburg," *British Medical Journal*, 29 (1975), pp. 489–493.

63. D. H. Smith, B. K. Johnson, and M. Isaacson, "Marburg Virus Disease in Kenya," *Lancet*, 1 (1982), pp. 816–820.

64. Tom Curtis, "The Origin of AIDS," *Rolling Stone*, 19 March 1992, pp. 54–61, 106.

65. See Thierry Huet, Remi Cheynier, Andreas Meyerhans, Georges Roelants, and Simon Wain–Hobson, "Genetic Organization of a Chimpanzee Lentivirus Related to HIV–1," *Nature*, 345 (1990), pp. 356–359; P.J. Kanki, J. Alroy, and M. Essex, "Isolation of T–Lymphotropic Retrovirus Related to HTLV–III/LAV from Wild–Caught African Green Monkeys," *Science* (1985), pp. 951–954; Lisa Chakrabarti, Mireille Guyader, Marc Alizon, Muthiah D. Daniel, Ronald C. Desrosiers, Pierre Tiollais, and Pierre Sonigo, "Sequence of Simian Immunodeficiency Virus from Macaque and Its Relationship to Other Human and Simian Viruses," *Nature*, 328 (1987), pp. 543–547.

66. Myron Essex, "Origins of AIDS," in Vincent T. DeVita, Samuel Hellman and Steven A. Rosenberg (eds.), *AIDS: Etiology, Siagnosis, Treatment, and Prevention* (Philadelphia: J.B. Lippincott, 1988), pp. 3–10.

67. R. C. Desrosiers and N. L. Letvin, "Animal Models for Acquired Immunodeficiency Syndrome," *Reviews of Infectious Diseases*, 9 (1987), pp. 438–446; M. B. Gardner and P. A. Luciw, "Simian Immunodeficiency Viruses and Their Relationship to Human Immunodeficiency Viruses," *AIDS*, 2, Supp. 1 (1988), pp. S3–S10.

68. Jon Cohen, "Debate on AIDS Origin: *Rolling Stone* Weighs In," *Science*, 255 (1992), p. 1505; Nancy Touchette, "Wistar Panel Disputes Polio Vaccine–HIV Link," *Journal of NIH Research*, 4 (1992), p. 42.

69. Quoted in Rutledge, p. 256.

70. James H. McNeill, "The Plague of Plagues," *New York Review of Books*, 21 July 1983, pp. 28–29.

71. Robert S. Gottfried, *The Black Death: Natural and Human Disaster in Medieval Europe* (New York: Free Press, 1983).

72. James Kinsella, *Covering the Plague: AIDS and the American Media* (New Brunswick, NJ: Rutgers University Press, 1989), p. 127.

73. Kinsella, p. 122.

74. Kinsella, p. 124.

75. Shilts, p. 175.

76. Altman, p. 26.

77. Kinsella, p. 280.

78. Larry Kramer, *Reports from the Holocaust: The Making of an AIDS Activist* (New York: St. Martin's Press, 1989), p. 149.

79. Kramer, pp. 159–160.

CHAPTER TWO

Contagious Desire: Sex, Drugs, Disease, and HIV

Thomas Robert Malthus, the early nineteenth-century economist, is generally considered to be the founder of population study as a field of scholarship. Since the publication in 1798 of the first edition of his *An Essay on the Principle of Population*, his views have been the subject of many heated discussions. Malthus asserted that human populations tended to increase at a more rapid rate than the food supply needed to sustain them. He had come to this conclusion on the basis of several postulates about peoples' material needs, sexual instincts, and reproductive capacities. His basic theory was stated in three distinct principles:

1. Population is necessarily limited to the means of subsistence.
2. Population invariably increases where the means of subsistence increases, unless prevented by some powerful and obvious checks.
3. These checks, and the checks which repress the superior power of population and keep its effects on a level with the means of subsistence, are all resolvable into moral restraint, vice, and misery.[1]

Propositions One and Two suggested that if population always increases to the point where any further increase is checked by the limits of the food supply, then material progress can generate no significant improvements in living conditions. Malthus was contending here that instead of permitting the existing population to lead a better life, increases in food production merely allowed a larger population to subsist at the same low level that prevailed prior to the increased food output. "Moral restraint," he added in Proposition Three, in the forms of "late marriage and abstinence (from sex) in marriage," was a positive check against population growth, but so too were "vice and misery" (war, infanticide, plague, and famine). There was more:

Assuming then, my postula as granted, I say, that the power of population is indefinitely greater than the power in the earth to produce subsistence for man. Population, when unchecked, increases in a geometrical ratio. Subsistence increases in only an arithmetical ratio.* A slight acquaintance with numbers will show the immensity of the first power in comparison with the second.[2]

When viewed from the vantage point of the late twentieth century, Malthus' theory reflects four significant weaknesses.[3] First, he placed undue emphasis on the limited amount of food that the land could yield. His predictions did not come about, at least in part, because of the nineteenth-century revolution in agricultural methods—crop rotation, chemical fertilizers, plant and animal breeding, and improved livestock feed. Many more scientific techniques were developed in the twentieth century in the areas of agriculture and animal reproduction, resulting in the ability of "subsistence," to use Malthus' term, to increase at a geometric rate.

Second, Malthus had the misfortune—from the standpoint of his theory—of writing on the eve of the Industrial Revolution. As such, he failed to recognize the possibilities for improvement in standards of living through industrialization, better methods of production and transportation, and superior distribution techniques. In short, he fully underestimated the potential for invention and innovation.

Third, and also related to industrialization, Malthus' argument did not take into consideration the faster and more reliable modes of transport that helped colonial empires to provide additional raw materials, an exploitable labor supply, and new markets for manufactured products. The emergence of a flourishing international trade and the outpouring of emigrants from Europe provided relief from population pressures in the home nations as well as the needed labor supply in the New World.

Fourth, and perhaps most importantly, Malthus had ignored the possibilities of birth control. His religious beliefs defined contraception as immoral, so he never gave consideration to its widespread use.

Immediately following the publication of his book in 1798, Malthus became the focus of intense controversy. Numerous written responses both supported and opposed his theory. Yet following his death in 1834, his theory quickly dropped from favor. By then, the Industrial Revolution had begun, and the vast grassy plains of North America had been opened to cultivation. The new lands and more efficient means of production and distribution had eliminated from people's thoughts the mass destitution that had given Malthus' doctrines meaning during his lifetime.

---

*Arithmetical ratios increase in the form of 1, 2, 3, 4, 5, 6, 7, and so forth. Geometrical ratios increase in the form of a geometric progression: 1, 2, 4, 8, 16, 32, 64, and so on.

Readers might be wondering at this point, "Why all this attention to Malthus? What does his disfavored eighteenth-century theory have to do with AIDS?" The issue is this: Malthus spoke of exponential growth, and many others have in the years hence. Remember the problem: if you place a penny on square one of a checkerboard and double the number of coins on each subsequent square—2, 4, 8, 16, 32. . .—how big is the stack by the 64th square? The answer: about as high as the universe is wide. After 10 steps, you have passed the thousandth mark; after 20 steps, the millionth mark. No system can survive very many steps of exponential growth. That was one of the problems of population increase contemplated by Malthus. Exponential growth has been similarly contemplated with respect to the spread of AIDS and its impact on population and society.[4]

THE EPIDEMIOLOGY OF AIDS

What was clear about AIDS from the outset was its exponential growth rate—eight cases prior to 1979, then 10 new cases in 1979, 46 more in 1980, another 252 in 1981, an so on, until by the close of the 1980s the number of diagnosed cases in the United States alone had accumulated to well over 100,000. It appeared, too, that once the virus invaded a population, it spread rapidly.

There were times when there was a "doubling" of known cases every five months, and it was then that people began to wonder where it would all end. Doomsday prophecies held that AIDS was nature's answer to overpopulation. Also, there were the arguments that the disease had been wrought by God to punish those who were infecting the world with sin.[5] There were many cruel and hostile jokes as well.* But as the demographers and other scientists who came after Malthus have learned, exponential growth in a finite world has its limits. It either destroys the entire system or the process slows down.

By 1987, in the United States at any rate, there did appear to be signs of a slowing—at least in terms of the doubling time (see Figure I). The numbers of newly diagnosed AIDS cases were still increasing rapidly, reaching an accumulated total of some 250,000 by the end of 1992.[6] But the doubling time had gone from five months early in the decade to 13 months five years later, and to 24 months by the early 1990s. As reflected in Figure II, the number of new AIDS cases in the United States increased dramatically, but this was a result of a new and more inclusive definition of what constituted AIDS.[7]

---

*In this regard, gay men were most often targets of the hostile joking. One of the many phrases to connect AIDS with biblical retribution was, "The new acronym for AIDS: WOGS—Wrath of God Syndrome."See David Black, *The Plague Years: A Chronicle of AIDS: The Epidemic of Our Times* (New York: Simon and Schuster, 1986), pp. 29-30.

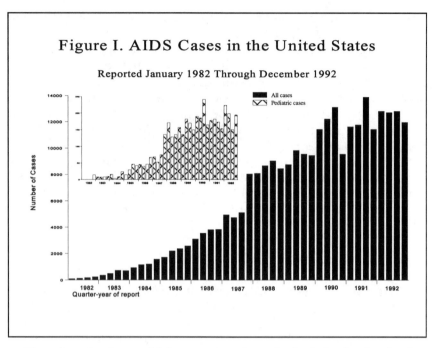

Figure I. AIDS Cases in the United States

Reported January 1982 Through December 1992

Elsewhere in the world, however, and particularly in the developing nations of Central and West Africa, a rather different picture was emerging. While the World Health Organization was reporting less than 12,000 AIDS cases on the entire African continent in mid-1988, the figure referred only to "known" *diagnosed* cases. Estimates as to the numbers of Africans infected with HIV were as high as 30 to 40 million.[8] By the close of 1992, it was estimated that upwards of 20 percent of the sexually active population in many nations in Sub-Saharan Africa were HIV positive.[9] And in parts of Asia and Latin America, rates were growing even more rapidly.

Within this context, and from analyses of AIDS reports and HIV testing data, it appears that there are at least four distinct patterns of AIDS across the globe.[10]

Pattern-I seems to be typical of industrialized nations with relatively large numbers of AIDS cases, such as the United States, Canada, Mexico, many Western European countries, and Australia and New Zealand (see Figure III). In Pattern-I nations, HIV probably began to spread extensively during the late 1970s. Most cases occur among men who have sex with men (homosexuals and bisexuals) and intravenous and other injection drug users.* Heterosexual transmission of the vi-

---

*A distinction is made here between "intravenous" and other "injection" drug users because there are alternative ways of injecting drugs. *Intravenous* (IV or "mainlining") use involves an injection directly into the vein. There is *intramuscular* or IM (into the muscle) injection, *intradermal* (into the skin), and *subcutaneous* (under the skin) injection.

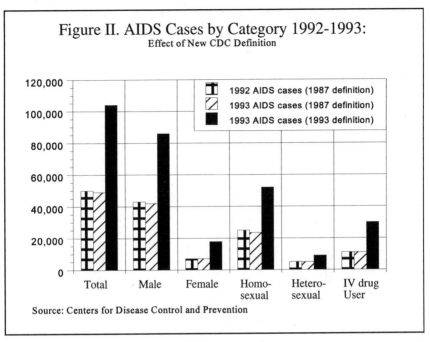

Figure II. AIDS Cases by Category 1992-1993:
Effect of New CDC Definition

Legend:
- 1992 AIDS cases (1987 definition)
- 1993 AIDS cases (1987 definition)
- 1993 AIDS cases (1993 definition)

Categories: Total, Male, Female, Homosexual, Heterosexual, IV drug User

Source: Centers for Disease Control and Prevention

rus, although markedly increasing, is responsible for only a small proportion of cases. There was transmission of HIV through some transfusions of blood and blood products in Pattern-I countries between the late 1970s and 1985. That route of transmission, however, has been practically eliminated in some countries and drastically reduced in others by the convincing of those at risk for HIV infection not to donate blood and by the testing of potential blood donors for the presence of HIV antibodies.[11] Unsterile needles, aside from those used by injection drug users, are not a significant factor in the transmission of HIV in Pattern-I nations. Finally, fewer women are infected in these countries, and, as a result, perinatal transmission (from mother to infant) is also low. Since heterosexual transmission is increasing, however, so too are HIV infections in women and infants. The current male-to-female ratio of reported AIDS cases in Pattern-I countries ranges from 10-to-1 to 15-to-1. But this is rapidly changing, due to the growing spread of the virus in populations of injection drug users and their sex partners.

Pattern-II can be observed in Haiti and other parts of the Caribbean, and much of Sub-Saharan Africa (see Figure IV). As in the Pattern-I nations, Pattern-II areas saw the initial spread of the virus during the late 1970s. Unique to this pattern, however, the male-to-female ratio is

---

Intramuscular, intradermal, and subcutaneous injections are sometimes referred to as "skinning," "skin popping," or just "popping."

Figure III. Pattern I Nations

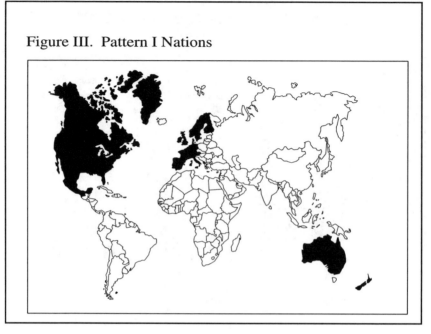

almost 1-to-1, with most cases occurring among heterosexuals. Transmission through male homosexual activity or injection drug use is either absent or at a low level, whereas perinatal transmission is common.

In the developing nations of Central and West Africa, the epidemic character of AIDS is related in part to existing health-care practices. Many such practices tend to be unsanitary; they include particularly the reuse of unsterilized hypodermic needles by local healers and, early in the AIDS epidemic, for transfusions in rural and bush hospitals and mass inoculations.[12] In addition, a strong link exists in this part of the world between AIDS and prostitution. As one observer explained the situation:

> A study of Nairobi's Kenyatta Hospital shows just how fast a virus can spread in a society where sexual partners change frequently. Within six years, 60 percent of all prostitutes examined were carriers (of HIV). In the slums of Nairobi today, there is almost no prostitute who is not infected with the virus. The women, most of whom were forced by poverty to leave their native villages, have about 1,000 customers a year. After spending a while in the slums, the women return to their families on the land. They bring the plague with them.[13]

An additional element in Africa concerns the fact that the disease has been compounded by other infections—malaria, yellow fever, tuberculosis, leprosy, and sexually transmitted diseases and by under-

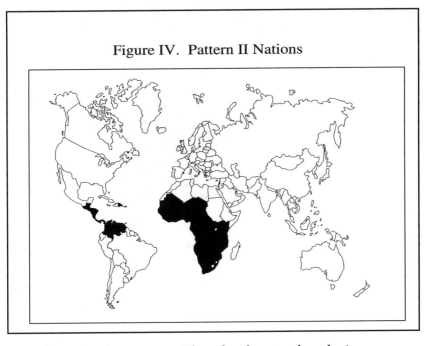

Figure IV. Pattern II Nations

nourishment and pregnancy. These burdens weaken the immune system, making it easier for HIV to establish itself.

During the early years of the AIDS epidemic, given the prevalence of AIDS among Haitian immigrants, the Centers for Disease Control classified them as a separate "risk group" for the disease. As pointed out in Chapter One, however, focused study of the Haitian cases in Miami and New York determined that *being Haitian* was not necessarily a risk factor for AIDS. Rather, as in Africa, there were other variables—prostitution, malnutrition, and a complex of sexually transmitted and other diseases that exposed the immunocompromised individual to more possibilities of infection.[14]

Pattern-III prevails in sections of Eastern Europe, North Africa, the Middle East, much of Asia, and the majority of the Pacific (see Figure V). In these areas, HIV was likely introduced during the early and mid-1980s. Only small numbers of cases have been observed, and these are primarily in people who have traveled to Pattern-I or Pattern-II countries and had sexual contacts during their visits. Indigenous homosexual, heterosexual, and injection drug transmission patterns have been documented only recently. Finally, some cases have been caused by imported blood products that were contaminated by HIV.

The principal reasons for the fewer numbers of cases in those Pattern-III countries formerly referred to as the Warsaw Bloc nations and the Union of Soviet Socialist Republics were under-reporting and re-

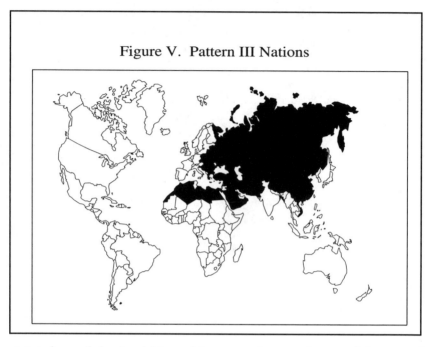

Figure V. Pattern III Nations

stricted travel, both within and between these nations and the rest of the world. As contact with the West increased, however, so too have HIV and AIDS.

Pattern-IV includes those nations in which the prevalence of HIV and AIDS has shifted from being predominantly among homosexual men to primarily heterosexuals and children (see Figure VI). In parts of Central and South America and the Caribbean basin, the introduction of HIV infection into the heterosexual population would appear to be more a function of bisexuality than injection drug use. Recent research in Brazil suggests this to be especially the case in parts of that country.[15] As such, it would appear that Brazil incorporates aspects of Patterns I and II, with a pattern of HIV infection from an initially male homosexual population to the larger heterosexual population by means of bisexuals.*

By contrast, what would appear to be a wholly unique pattern was uncovered in Rumania during the early weeks of 1990. After the fall of dictator Nicolae Ceausescu, Western physicians revealed a mysterious epidemic of AIDS among segments of Rumania's infant population housed in hospitals and orphanages. Two theories were posed to explain the phenomenon. The first related to the traditional practice in Rumania of injecting minute quantities of adult blood into infants who

_____

*AIDS and its relation to the sexual culture in Brazil are discussed at length in Chapter Four of this book.

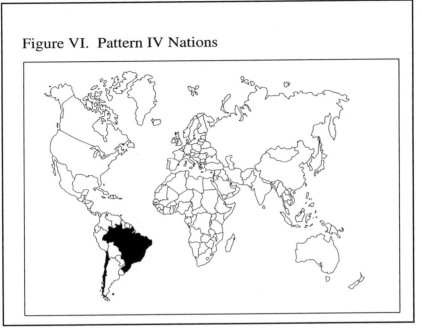

Figure VI. Pattern IV Nations

appeared anemic. The blood supply used for this purpose was likely contaminated. The second pathway of infection was from the reuse of dirty needles. As was the case in most Eastern European countries at the time, disposable syringes were in short supply, and hospital staff were not always trained properly in effective sterilizing techniques.[16]

Prior to the fall of Ceausescu, Rumania was considered a low-risk country. As of December 31, 1989, it had officially reported only 13 AIDS cases to the World Health Organization. Due to the lack of hard currency, trafficking in such expensive drugs as heroin and cocaine was not a problem. Male homosexuality did not appear to be an important factor in the spread of HIV. Moreover, homosexual acts among consenting adults were forbidden by law, punishable by sentences of imprisonment of up to five years.[17] But by February 9, 1990, 706 children with HIV were found in the cities of Bucharest, Constanta, Guirgiu, Focsani, and Arad. Half of the 200 children tested in Constanta orphanages were HIV positive. By the close of 1990, there were 1,168 known AIDS cases in Rumania, of which 94 percent were infants and children under the age of 4 at the time of diagnosis, and the majority of these were abandoned children living in public institutions.[18]

In 1992, the World Health Organization estimated that as many as 10 million people around the globe were infected with HIV, and that 40 million would be infected by the end of the century.[19] In 1994, the World Health Organization reaffirmed this estimate.[20] Although het-

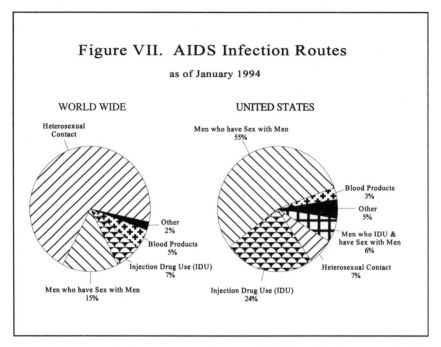

Figure VII. AIDS Infection Routes

as of January 1994

WORLD WIDE

Heterosexual Contact

Other 2%

Blood Products 5%

Injection Drug Use (IDU) 7%

Men who have Sex with Men 15%

UNITED STATES

Men who have Sex with Men 55%

Blood Products 3%

Other 5%

Men who IDU & have Sex with Men 6%

Heterosexual Contact 7%

Injection Drug Use (IDU) 24%

erosexual transmission accounts for much of the infection worldwide, in the United States those dominating the AIDS caseload include men who have sex with men, followed by injection drug users (see Figure VII). The issues associated with the transmission of HIV and AIDS are addressed at length in the sections that follow.

GAY MEN AND SAME-SEX RISK BEHAVIORS

Just after midnight on June 27, 1969, nine plainclothes police detectives entered the Stonewall Inn at 53 Christopher Street in New York's *avant garde* Greenwich Village. The Stonewall was an unlicensed gay bar, and the intentions of the detectives were to close it down. Such raids were routine enough, but on that particular night the atmosphere at the Stonewall was jubilant. When a few of the club's occupants emerged in police custody, a growing mob of mainly gay and transvestite onlookers cheered them on. "We're the Pink Panthers" and "I like boys," some jeered, and a mobile chorus of transvestites mocked the police with an impromptu cancan.

As the crowd expanded to almost 400, they began throwing coins, bottles, and bricks. The officers retreated into the Stonewall, but someone found a parking meter and thrust it through the door. Others shouted "Pigs!" and "Faggot cops!" A burning garbage can was also hurled inside. As police reinforcements arrived, the crowd began to disperse, and the 45-minute riot was suddenly over.[21]

On the following night there was a second riot in Greenwich Village. As a crowd gathered outside the Stonewall Inn to protest the previous night's raid, police tactical units poured into the area. Many of the protesters did little more than shout slogans—"Legalize gay bars!" "Gay is good!"—and one group chanted:

> We are the Stonewall girls.
> We wear our hair in curls.
> We have no underwear.
> We show our pubic hair![22]

Others in the crowd were not quite as controlled—throwing rocks and setting fires. After two hours of uproar and chaos, police armed with billy clubs charged and dispersed the mob. On June 29th only a brief report of the confrontations appeared on one of the back pages of *The New York Times*, entitled "Four Policemen Hurt in 'Village' Raid."[23]

On July 2nd there was yet another protest. According to one eyewitness, the police, armed with night sticks, seemed bent on retaliation:

> At one point, Seventh Avenue looked like a battlefield in Vietnam. Young people, many of them queens, were lying on the sidewalk, bleeding from the head, face, mouth, and even the eyes.[24]

"Stonewall," as these events have come to be known, was significant in the fight for gay liberation. Although the raid did not mark the beginning of the gay rights movement, it did mark a generational and ideological shift that brought gay liberation into the vast array of social protest first sparked by the sixties generation. Not surprisingly, the event received little media attention; even in the major chronicles of the 1960s Stonewall is never mentioned.[25] In Gay America, however, it had an immediate and seismic impact. Within days, activists formed the Gay Liberation Front, and a year later thousands of lesbians and gay men marched to celebrate the first anniversary of Stonewall.

As the gay liberation movement grew and prospered, the taverns and pubs buried in basements where many homosexuals had previously gathered were replaced with more well-kept gay bars and lounges. A side of the gay movement advocated promiscuity and the commercialization of gay sex in the form of bathhouses and sex clubs. Segments of this ethos of indiscriminate promiscuity was captured by gay writer Charley Shively in a controversial article written during the summer of 1974. Among other ideas, Shively asserted:

> We need to be more *promiscuous* as well as less discriminating. Promiscuous in every way with our bodies. Release all the armors and shackles, open all the pores and holes up for sexual communication. No restraint

in any way. Multiple loves—ameba-like as in orgies at the baths—single couplings, perhaps between subway stops or between classes or on the way shopping. We must be open at all times for sexual activity; in fact not make it an in-between action, but making every action sexual. Unlike capitalist decadence, our sexuality would not be separated from our business, our sexuality would not "drag" us down or wear us out for the tasks of building a totally free society. Our sexuality would be that society.[26]

Some gay men adopted the ideals and behavior extolled by Shively, and, from a medical standpoint, the promiscuity and the bathhouses were breeding grounds for disease. In addition to the more common sexually transmitted conditions as syphilis, gonorrhea, and hepatitis B, many gay men suffered from a range of parasitic infections of the colon, known collectively as the "gay bowel syndrome."[27] Unmistakably, many in the male gay community were vulnerable to the introduction of new sexually transmitted diseases.

Modes of HIV Transmission Among Gay Men

Among men who have sex with other men, HIV infection can be transmitted in two basic ways—sexually and through direct contact with infected blood. Gay and bisexual men generally acquire HIV infection through sexual contact, and the risk of acquisition of infection depends on two variables: 1) the probability of exposure to an infected partner; and, 2) the probability of transmission from the infected partner.

The first variable, that sexual contact with a person known to be infected with HIV is associated with transmission, has been well documented.[28] There is ample epidemiologic evidence that during homosexual intercourse, the virus is transmitted from the penis of the insertive partner into the anus and rectum of the receptive partner. Insertive anal intercourse confers risk as well, but the magnitude of that risk has been difficult to establish. As the prevalence of HIV has increased, the probability that a randomly chosen sex partner is infected has also increased. All things considered, the risk for exposure per contact in 1994 is substantially higher for homosexual men than it was a decade ago.

As with other sexually transmitted diseases, frequency of *unprotected* (without a condom) sexual contacts with numerous partners is likely the most important factor in the continued spread of HIV and AIDS among gay men. Recall the discussion in Chapter One of the case control study by the Centers for Disease Control in the early stages of the epidemic.[29] It was unprotected sex with a multiplicity of sex partners that was most strongly associated with risk. This finding was replicated in the San Francisco Men's Health Study in a cohort recruited during the latter part of 1984 from 19 census tracts where the

AIDS epidemic appeared to be most intense. In a representative sample of 796 homosexual men, the prevalence of HIV infection was approximately 18 percent among those who had only one or no sex partners during the prior two years, 32 percent in those reporting two to nine partners, 54 percent in those reporting 10 to 49 partners, and 71 percent in those reporting 50 or more partners.[30]

The second variable, the risk of effective transfer of the virus, is not quite as easy to assess, for it depends on the specific sexual practices and whether the virus in the body fluid of the infected donor comes into contact with an available receptor cell in the recipient. What is clear, however, is that almost all sexual acts may transmit the virus. In some of the major studies of prevalent HIV infection, unprotected receptive anal intercourse has been the major mode of transmission when other risk factors, including numbers of sex partners, were controlled for.[31] Similarly, unprotected receptive anal intercourse has been shown to be the primary mode of transmission of HIV in all cohort studies in which seroconversion* has been analyzed during follow-up.[32] There is the potential for HIV to be transmitted during oral-genital sex, but the findings in this area remain inconclusive.**

In addition to receptive anal intercourse, there are two other modes of HIV transmission among homosexual men, both involving the direct transfer of infected blood. The first is associated with blood transfusion, but few of these cases have been reported. The second involves the sharing of infected drug paraphernalia among gay men who are also injection drug users. As of early 1993, only 6 percent of all reported AIDS cases in the United States fell into this category.[33] Nevertheless, although the percentage may be small, the numbers are significant—almost 20,000—particularly since men who have sex with men who are also injection drug users represent a link in the chain of infection or "bridging group" to heterosexual populations.***

Cofactors for HIV Infection Among Gay Men

"Cofactors" include any physical conditions, behavioral practices, or microbiological agents that facilitate the transmission of HIV. Two major categories of cofactors have been investigated: 1) those that might affect acquisition of HIV before or during sexual contact (such as foreplay and other ancillary sexual practices); and 2) those of a more general nature having the potential to enhance susceptibility.

---

*The term *seroconversion* refers to the initial development of antibodies after contact with HIV. In other words, it is the shift from HIV-negative to HIV-positive.

**The potential for HIV transmission during oral sex is addressed in Chapter Four of this book.

***Drug injection practices are addressed at length later in this chapter.

There are two types of ancillary sexual practices among homosexual men of interest here, including:

- those that are likely to disrupt the sensitive tissues in the rectum, thereby facilitating infection; and

- those interfering with judgment that might render sex partners less likely to take precautions against acquiring infection.

The anus is a sensitive area, which, apart from its proximity to the genitals, appears to be intimately involved in both eliciting and responding to sexual stimuli. Some people react to anal stimulation erotically; others are indifferent to it or find it repugnant. Anal stimulation is not an exclusively male homosexual practice, for it occurs in heterosexual relations as well. In fact, in some cultures it is quite common as an alternative to vaginal intercourse.[34] The significant factor is that the tissues inside the rectum are highly delicate, and minor tearing of these sensitive membranes is possible during any form of anal intercourse. Even when lubricants are used, extremely vigorous intercourse can cause rectal trauma. Moreover, not uncommon during sexual activity is the insertion of fingers and dildos into the rectum, a practice that heightens the potential for trauma.

Data from the San Francisco Men's Health Study has documented that enemas and douching before sexual contact increase the risk of HIV infection during receptive anal intercourse.[35] For some gay men, the idea of having a sex partner administer an enema is exciting; for others, douching is intended for hygienic reasons. Those who tend toward enemas and douching find a variety of sizes, shapes, and forms of enema tubes available in stores that sell sexual products. The liquids that are utilized vary from warm water (with or without soap), to coffee or soft drinks, or even a sex partner's urine. In terms of exotica, one informant from Miami's Coconut Grove reported:

> I've done a lot of experimenting, with everything from cheap berry wine to olive oil. Seltzer is good too, but the best is a fine champagne, served at room temperature. Between the liquid, the bubbly, and the alcohol, it's a real rectal buzz.*

The problem with enemas and douching is the potential for rectal trauma. The findings of a large-scale study of risk factors for STD infection in gay men attending five public health clinics were consistent with observations of an association between douching and hepatitis B virus (HBV) infection.[36] Specifically, men who practiced rectal douching in association with passive anal-genital intercourse were found to be at greater risk for HBV infection. One can logically speculate that if this practice provides both a source of HBV infectious blood and a

---

*Douching with alcoholic beverages has potential hazards since absorption of drugs through rectal tissues is rapid.

portal of entry for HBV infection, the same would be the case for HIV infection.

An even greater likelihood for rectal injury exists with "fisting"—anal penetration by the fist, and sometimes by the forearm as well, through the rectum and possibly into the sigmoid colon.[37] A sharp fingernail can leave a deep cut in the rectum that can take weeks to heal. A fist ramming into the sigmoid colon—a part of the intestine several inches up from the anus—is even more problematic. The tissue lining the sigmoid colon has the consistency and delicacy of wet paper towels. In some people, the area can expand to accommodate a fist. Bleeding can result, and infection is likely.* With respect to enhancing HIV susceptibility through fisting, one observer of the gay scene recalled:

> By 1984, it was clear that AIDS was the result of some microbe—HIV, and possibly other agents as well—that could be transmitted via blood or semen. Yet what, it was asked, could possibly be transmitted from the fist to the rectum so long as the fist was clean or, at least, gloved in rubber? Researchers answered that inappropriate objects inserted into the rectum could cause abrasions or fissures through which HIV could later enter. But by the same logic, a mishap during *any* anal sex could also result in cuts and abrasions that, if the area were later exposed to blood or semen, could lead to HIV infection.[38]

As is the case with rectal douching, fisting has been found to be significantly related to HBV infection.[39]

Practices that interfere with judgment which might render sex partners less likely to take precautions against acquiring infection revolve around the use of psychoactive drugs. The most significant three drugs are the nitrite inhalants, alcohol, and cocaine.

The nitrites—principally amyl and butyl nitrite—are liquid compounds that were first introduced into medicine more than a century ago for the treatment of angina (heart pain). They have had other therapeutic uses as muscle relaxants and vasodilators (for increasing blood flow through capillaries). The primary effect of these drugs is to relax all of the smooth muscles in the body, including those in the blood vessels. They thus permit a greater flow of oxygenated blood to the brain.[40] Amyl and butyl nitrite were originally supplied in glass vials (ampules) which were broken open (or popped or snapped open) and inhaled, and hence, they were given such street names as "poppers"

---

*Readers may recall the arrest of a Cincinnati museum director in 1990 for exhibiting Robert Maplethorpe photographs. Subsequently there were "obscenity" and "indecency" restrictions placed on funding from the National Endowment for the Humanities (*The New York Times*, 7 Oct. 1990. p. 19; *The New York Times*, 20 Sept. 1991, p. B2). One of the Maplethorpe photographs to cause the most concern was his 1978 work, *Helmut and Brooks*, which was a depiction of "fisting." For a reproduction and discussion of *Helmut and Brooks* (and other Maplethorpe works), see Richard D. Mohr, *Gay Ideas: Outing and Other Controversies* (Boston: Beacon Press, 1992), pp. 188-189.

and "snappers." They are quick-acting drugs, taking effect in 15 to 30 seconds, with a duration of two to three minutes. On inhalation, there is a distinct "rush" (the initial flood of pleasure, with quickened heart rate, felt soon after the ingestion of certain psychoactive drugs).

The recreational popularity of the nitrites results from their reputation as aphrodisiacs. To gain this effect, they are usually inhaled just prior to orgasm. According to some observers, however, the reported intensification and prolongation of orgasm may be an illusion. The rush, involving dizziness and giddiness, may cause a reduction of social and sexual inhibitions along with time distortion. Clearly, this combination may lead to a sense of prolonged orgasm.[41] Some believe that an increased flow of blood to the genitals may indeed increase sensitivity to sexual activity.

For years, the nitrites were sold over the counter, but reports of widespread abuse during the 1960s resulted in their reclassification as prescription drugs. Since that time, however, other volatile nitrites containing isomers of amyl and butyl alcohol and butyl nitrite (unregulated by the Food and Drug Administration) have been marketed as "room deodorizers" and sold in bottles of 10 to 30 ml. Since their labels stated that they were not to be inhaled, they were legally sold, typically in pornographic and "head" shops, and through the mails under such names as *Hardware, Locker Room, Bolt, Rush,* and *Heart On.* Effective February 25, 1991, as an outgrowth of the 1990 Omnibus Crime Bill, the United States Senate banned the manufacture and sale of many nitrite products. Since then, however, a cyclohexyl nitrite has emerged that is being used as an inhalant.[42]

As noted earlier, the nitrites have been associated with the sexual activities of homosexual men more than with any other group (although they are used nonsexually as well, in discos and other dance clubs). Their popularity was related not only to their reputation as aphrodisiacs, but more realistically, to their ability to relax the sphincter (the bowel muscle), thus facilitating anal intercourse. In the early part of the AIDS epidemic, researchers at the National Institutes of Health suspected that nitrites might be immunosuppressive in the presence of repeated viral infections.[43] However, the findings of studies in this regard have been contradictory.[44] Nevertheless, the euphoria engendered from the nitrites can indeed interfere with good judgment, rendering some users less likely to take precautions against acquiring infection. As one informant reported to the authors:

> Amyl nitrite and condoms don't go together. When I'm on a high rush and my dick is hard, I'm not thinking about rubbers, just fucking and getting off.

In the early years of the epidemic, the use of nitrites by gay men was suspected (and later dismissed) as a causative agent for AIDS. More recently, however, there has been speculation that the abuse of these drugs may be a cofactor in AIDS-related Kaposi's sarcoma (KS). In 1990, Dr. Harry W. Haverkos of the National Institute on Drug Abuse offered this suggestion for several reasons:

1. AIDS-related KS is more common among homosexual men than other risk groups and nitrite inhalants are used more commonly by gay men than others;

2. epidemiologic studies have shown a strong statistical association between the development of KS among homosexual men with AIDS and the use of large quantities of nitrite inhalants when compared with homosexual men with AIDS but without KS; and,

3. anecdotal reports of the increased frequency of AIDS-related KS on the face and chest, and especially the nose, are consistent with the likely areas of skin most heavily exposed to nitrite vapors when inhaled.[45]

Alcohol's relationship to high-risk sexual behavior has been well documented. In several studies of homosexual men, for example, alcohol use combined with sexual activity was found to be strongly associated with such risky practices as receptive anal intercourse, multiple anonymous sex partners, and lack of condom use.[46] Cocaine has long since had a reputation for being a spectacular aphrodisiac; it is believed to create sexual desire, to heighten it, to increase sexual endurance, and to cure frigidity and impotence.[47]

One of the more interesting investigations of psychoactive drug use and risky behaviors among gay men was initiated in New York City during 1985.[48] A sample of 746 gay men were recruited for an assessment of the social and psychological impact of the AIDS epidemic on the local gay community. The inclusion criteria were a) having a gay or bisexual orientation, b) being 18 years or older, and c) residing in New York City. The only exclusion criterion was having a diagnosis of AIDS. There were two subsequent interviews at one-year intervals, in 1986 and 1987, and men who failed to complete all three interviews or who developed AIDS during the course of the study were not included in the drug use/sexual risk analysis. The final sample of 604 men were questioned about their drug using and sexual behaviors during four separate time periods: 1980–1981, 1984–1985, 1985–1986, and 1986–1987. In these data, the 1980–1981 time period represents the 12 months prior to the respondents' first learning about AIDS.

As indicated in Table 1, there were major changes within this population of gay men in the frequency of *unprotected* (without a condom) intercourse over the course of the study period. Whereas the members of the sample engaged in an average of 72.3 episodes of unprotected receptive anal intercourse and 77.6 episodes of unprotected insertive anal intercourse prior to hearing about AIDS, these averages dropped to 5.6 and 6.1, respectively, by the 1986–1987 period.

TABLE 1: Drug Use and Anal Intercourse Among Gay Men

	Average Annual Frequency of Engaging in Unprotected Anal Intercourse Among Final Panel Sample Members			
		Year		
Type of Anal Intercourse	1980–81	1984–85	1985–86	1986–87
Receptive	72.3	16.5	7.1	5.6*
	(209.5)	(39.3)	(23.1)	(27.9)
Insertive	77.6	20.9	10.3	6.1*
	(153.0)	(47.4)	(29.8)	(22.5)

Notes. N = 604; standard deviations are in parentheses.
*p .0001 (1980–1981 vs. 1986–1987).

Source: Adapted from John L. Martin, "Drug Use and Unprotected Anal Intercourse Among Gay Men," *Health Psychology*, 9 (1990), pp. 450–465.

Table 2 reflects the frequency of drug use during sex. Although the data document that the proportions of gay men using specific drugs declined as the AIDS epidemic unfolded, significant levels of drug use nevertheless persisted. More importantly, however, analyses found that unprotected anal sex, even in the more recent stages of the epidemic, occurred more often when the participants in the episode were under the influence of drugs.

TABLE 2: Drug Use and Anal Intercourse Among Gay Men

	Proportion of Final Panel Sample Members Using Drugs With Sex			
		Year		
Drug Use	1980–81	1984–85	1985–86	1986–87
Marijuana	.60	.45	.39	.33
Inhaled nitrite	.59	.42	.32	.25
Cocaine	.19	.22	.16	.14
Hallucinogen	.18	.09	.08	.06
Barbiturate	.16	.05	.03	.02
Amphetamine	.12	.04	.04	.01
Any drug	.73	.60	.52	.45

Notes. N = 604; all 1986–1987 proportions are significantly lower than 1980–1981 proportions based on t tests for correlated proportional differences: p .01 after applying Bonferroni inequality for multiple significance tests.

Source: Adapted from John L. Martin, "Drug Use and Unprotected Anal Intercourse Among Gay Men," *Health Psychology*, 9 (1990), pp. 450–465.

There is a rather wide range of concurrent or prior infections that represent cofactors of a more general nature which have the potential to enhance susceptibility to HIV. Of most significance are infections associated with enteric and sexually transmitted diseases. Syphilis, gonorrhea, and anal and genital warts and herpes have been associated with HIV infection. Then there are the enteric diseases—particularly amebiasis, giardiasis, and shigella—which are caused by organisms that lodge themselves in the intestinal tracts of gay men. Such infections are typically the result of anal intercourse, which puts an individual in contact with his partner's fecal matter. An even more direct mechanism of ingesting the parasitic spoor associated with these conditions comes from the practice of "rimming" (oral-anal intercourse)— the act of placing one's tongue into the anus of another.[49] Or in the more precise language of medical science:

> Sexual transmission of enteric pathogens which are shed in feces may be attributable to ingestion of feces during anilingus or during fellation of a fecally contaminated penis or to direct intrarectal inoculation of organisms by a fecally contaminated penis.[50]

The resulting parasitic infections often cause chronic diarrhea, which can bring on significant immune suppression.[51] These parasitic infections pose yet another immunosuppressive risk for gay men, for many antiparasitic drugs can have adverse effects on the immune system. Decreased immune response, furthermore, increases one's susceptibility to HIV infection.

Interestingly, in the beginning of the AIDS epidemic when the etiology of the disease was still a matter of intense speculation, there was a search for risk factors that seemed to be common to the gay community but less frequently found in other populations. The most obvious among these was anal intercourse, and a second was the use of nitrite inhalants, as already noted above. There was also a third factor. During the second half of the 1970s, at a time when HIV and AIDS were acronyms unknown by medical science, the male gay community was facing a relatively new and puzzling malady that came to be known as (and misnamed) the "gay bowel syndrome."[52] Although the condition had been recognized as early as 1968,[53] it did not appear to be a major problem until a decade later. During the period 1978 through 1982, for example, the San Francisco Department of Health reported a tenfold increase in cases of intestinal parasites in men ages 20 to 39 years.[54] Subsequently, a temporal relationship was found between the emergence of the epidemic of intestinal parasites in homosexual men and the subsequent appearance of Kaposi's sarcoma.[55] As such, and as has been speculated with nitrite inhalants, perhaps there is an association between the presence of intestinal parasites and the development of Kaposi's sarcoma.

The Natural History of HIV Infection in Homosexual Men

The natural history of HIV infection can be divided into three stages—the primary stage, extending from the time of infection through seroconversion; the secondary stage, from seroconversion through the onset of AIDS; and the tertiary stage, from the diagnosis of AIDS until death.[56] With regard to the primary stage, several studies have attempted to establish the probable time between exposure to HIV and seroconversion. Early in the epidemic, the consensus of opinion was that the typical time between transmission of the virus and sero-conversion was six to eight weeks, but with the recognition that detection of antibodies might not occur until eight months after an isolated exposure to HIV.[57] More recently, while a few investigations have suggested incubation periods of one to two weeks and three to 14 days,[58] others have found ranges of six to 56 days and eight to 10 weeks.[59] What is clear is that the period of incubation is highly variable, with the divergence most likely dependent on the amount of viral particles a person is exposed to, the form in which they are transmitted, and the condition of the immune system.

The time between seroconversion resulting from sexual contact between homosexual men and the onset of AIDS—the secondary stage—is generally long and also quite variable. In one study of homosexual men whose seroconversion dates were known, 30 percent had developed AIDS over an average follow-up of 76 months, and between 26 percent and 46 percent developed AIDS within 88 months.[60] Among homosexual men in general, presumably infected through sexual contact, the onset of AIDS has been observed as soon as 12 months and as long as eight years after seroconversion.[61]

The tertiary stage in the natural history of HIV infection in homosexual men is relatively short. The deteriorating clinical status of AIDS patients is characterized by severe wasting, protracted diarrhea, high fevers, and respiratory complications associated with a wide variety of opportunistic infections, and severe neurological disorders and central nervous system complications. To date, no one has recovered from this tertiary stage of HIV infection, and the final days are often painful and lonesome. As Steven Petrow of the San Francisco AIDS Foundation wrote in his journal on May 5, 1987:

> I went to see Eddie today after finding out yesterday that he had pneu-mocystis again. His voice on the phone was rough and sounded tired, but he made sense. I was unprepared for what I saw today. In fact, I realized I was unprepared to deal with the reality of his death.
>
> Eddie could not speak. He could hardly breathe. His legs were covered with the grotesque purple lesions. So were his arms and his chest and his belly. They were everywhere, and they were overwhelming. A cancer

was consuming him. No metaphors, no nothing. He was rotting. What could be inside him?

It is difficult to write what it is like to be with someone who is dying from AIDS. His eyes remained closed as noises reverberated deep inside. Suddenly, his body would spasm; then it would lie quiet again.

> He seemed to be crying.
> He was out of his mind.
> His pain was immense.
> And he was alone.[62]

HIV, AIDS, AND INJECTION DRUG USERS

In late 1984, at a time when the number of known AIDS cases in the United States was just below 8,000, a 38-year-old Miami heroin user, known on the street as Henry J., commented to one of the authors:

AIDS? What's that? I don't know what you're talkin' about. Wasn't that, isn't that, just some kind of . . . a gum, diet gum, or candy, or something like that?My old lady was into that once.

. . . A disease? FTS [fuck that shit]! Don't go givin' me another story 'bout why it's bad shootin' up. Don't want any more of your social worker crapola shit.

Less than two years later, as of April 4, 1986, physicians and health departments across the United States had notified the Centers for Disease Control of 19,181 AIDS cases—18,907 adults and 274 children—of whom 10,152 had already died. Some 17 percent of the total cases were injection drug users. Later that month, Henry J., by then age 40 and just moving into his twenty-second consecutive year of intravenous drug use, offered the following observation:

Hey, I heard of yer disease. I seen Dan Rather talk 'bout it on the news. Some kind of fuckin' homo disease mainly, goddamn ass fuckers, but ya can get it from shootin' up too, so I hear, if you're not careful.

Right? But hell. What else is new, tell me what else is new, will ya? I told ya once that you're not a man until you've had a good dose of the clap [gonorrhea] at least a few times. Well, same thing goes. What kind of a dope fiend are ya if ya haven't been to the ER [emergency room] a few times—an OD [overdose], hepatitis, AIDS—so what's the difference? I been to the big "J" [Miami's Jackson Memorial Hospital] all kinds of times, you know, and for all kinds of things. Ha, and even for the clap once. So what's the big deal? If I get it [AIDS] I'll deal with it then.

Six months later Henry J. noted:

So OK 'bout your AIDS stuff. It's more serious than the clap. OK, OK! People, some of 'em anyway, are bein' more careful. Some of 'em rinse their needles better. And me, I don't shoot up now with anyone I don't know, or didn't run with before, especially if they look sick.[63]

In January, 1987, after entering a drug treatment program under a court order, Henry J. tested positive for HIV. By Thanksgiving he had experienced several bouts with, among other ailments, *P-carinii* pneumonia. On December 31, 1987, Henry J. died of AIDS while being taken by ambulance to Miami's Jackson Memorial Hospital. A few months later, his sister recalled:

> Because of his drug use, Henry was always getting sick, but nothing ever like this. Thinking back, it began as just minor things—he lost a few pounds, then coughing, fevers on and off, things like that. Some days he'd be real weak, other days he seemed fine. None of us thought about AIDS. But then things really got bad. In his last few months, Henry kept getting pneumonia, he had herpes, problems with his kidneys, and all kinds of really strange infections that none of us understood. Then he got TB, and his body just seemed to melt away. By the time he died, he was only 92 pounds. And what most people didn't know was that when he died, he was blind, too.

HIV Transmission Among Injection Drug Users

The sharing of hypodermic needles, syringes, and other injection equipment is the most likely route of HIV transmission among intravenous and other injection drug users. The vector is the exchange of the blood of the previous user that is lodged in the needle, the syringe, or some other part of the *works* (drug paraphernalia).

Levels of risk vary, however, depending on the particular injection practice. Of lesser risk, for example, is *skin-popping*—the intradermal (into the skin), subcutaneous (under the skin), or intramuscular (into the muscle) injection of cocaine, narcotics, and other drugs. Skin-popping (or simply *popping*) is a common method of heroin use by experimenters and *tasters* (novice and casual users) who mistakenly believe that addiction cannot occur through this route.[64]

At the opposite end of the risk spectrum is *booting*, a process involving the use of a syringe to draw blood from the user's arm, the mixing of the drawn blood with the drug already taken into the syringe, and the injection of the blood/drug mixture into the vein. Many injection drug users believe that this practice potentiates a drug's effects. Importantly, however, booting leaves traces of blood in the needle and syringe, thus placing subsequent users of the injection equipment at risk.[65] Although most injection drug users are generally aware of the risks associated with booting and needle sharing, the risks are often ignored. Moreover, little thought is typically given to the risks associated with other aspects of the injection process.

Virological studies have indicated that HIV can survive in ordinary tap water for extended periods of time. In a series of experiments conducted at the Laboratory of Tumor Cell Biology, National Institutes of Health, for example, infectious cell-free virus could be recovered from dried material after up to three days at room temperature. In an aqueous medium, viruses survived longer than 15 days at room temperature.[66] Similar results were found in complementary studies conducted at the Institute Pasteur in Paris.[67] Along comparable lines, researchers at the University of Miami School of Medicine demonstrated the viability of HIV in blood and cell culture medium in needles and syringes at room temperatures for up to 24 hours.[68] The implication of these findings is that shared water used in the injection process represents a potential disease reservoir.

Injection drug users require water both to rinse their syringes and to mix with their drugs to liquefy them for injection. Rinsing, for example, is not necessarily for hygienic purposes, but to make sure a syringe does not become clogged with blood and drug residue, so that it can be used again. This rinse water is often shared. As one user explained:

> People don't clean their works before they shoot dope, they clean them afterward, and they clean them out of the same cup of water that everyone is using. So, while somebody is rinsing their syringe out in a cup of water, another person is pulling water out into their spoon to cook their dope in.[69]

As such, water contaminated through the rinsing of a syringe is used for rinsing other syringes and for mixing the drug. Similarly, *spoons, cookers,* and *cottons* are parts of the injection kit that also represent potential reservoirs of disease. Spoons and cookers are the bottle caps, spoons, baby-food jars, and other small containers used for mixing the drug, while cottons refer to any materials placed in the spoon to filter out undissolved drug particles. Filtering is considered necessary since undissolved particles tend to clog injection equipment. The risks of HIV infection from spoons and cottons are due to their frequent sharing, even by drug users who carry their own syringes.

Viral contamination might also result from *frontloading* and *backloading,* techniques for distributing a drug solution among a drug injecting group.[70] When frontloading, the drug is transferred from the syringe used for measuring by removing the needle from the receiving syringe and squirting the solution directly into its hub. Common in Miami "shooting galleries"* is the intercontamination of drug doses through the mixing and frontloading of *speedball* (heroin and cocaine).

---

*Shooting galleries are one of many kinds of places where drugs are used and/or shared, and are discussed at length in Chapter Three of this book.

Since heroin is "cooked" (heated in an aqueous solution) during its preparation for injecting but cocaine is not, separate containers are used for the mixing process. Those who share speedball draw the heroin into one syringe and the cocaine into another, remove the needle from the cocaine syringe and discharge the heroin into it through its hub, and return half the speedball mixture back into the syringe that originally contained the heroin. If either syringe contains virus at the start of such an operation, both are likely to contain it afterward.[71]

The backloading of speedball has also been observed in Miami galleries. Backloading involves essentially the same process, but the plunger, rather than the needle, is removed from the receiving syringe. Frontloading seems to be the preferred mixing/sharing method, with backloading as a substitute when syringes with detachable needles are unavailable.

Both frontloading and backloading have been reported by inmate informants in Delaware, Florida, New York, Maryland, and Ohio penitentiaries.[72] Illicit drugs are generally available in most American prisons, but typically in limited quantities and at considerable cost, often resulting in the sharing of injectable heroin, cocaine, and speedball by groups of three to four prisoners. Backloading is the preferred mixing/measuring technique. Since hypodermic syringes are closely controlled in prisons, makeshift injection equipment is manufactured from securable materials. A common "works" in the penitentiary is an eye dropper, with the glass or plastic end sharpened to an angular point. Backloading is accomplished by removing the squeeze bulb. Regarding the practice, an inmate in Miami's Dade County Stockade indicated in 1989:

> There's times when a backloaded dose is all you can get, with drugs bein' so scarce and all inside. They'll be someone with some dope and a few droppers with sharpened ends. You get your share by havin' yours pointed down with your finger covering the tip while someone loads it in.

An alternative method of drug sharing is referred to by some drug injectors as *shooting back* and *drawing up*. This practice has been observed in instances when every member of the drug-sharing group has a syringe. After the heroin, cocaine, or speedball is thoroughly mixed, it is discharged from the mixing syringe into a common spoon, cap, or container. Each member of the sharing group then draws a specific amount. As a former Delaware inmate described it:

> You see, when you're in that kind of situation you just have to make do. You just got to behave like some third world junkie who don't got either good drugs or good works. So you put together what everybody has, and you mix it, and then each one takes a turn to draw his share into the syringe.

But since we're not just third world junkies, we have etiquette—certain rules to follow. Like you don't shoot up until everyone's done drawing, because you got to see if it's shared equal. And sometimes there's arguments, because there's a motherfucker in the group who takes a little extra and tries to get away with it.

All forms of drug and equipment sharing tend to occur among *running partners* (or *running buddies*), drug users who are lovers, good friends, crime partners, or live together. They serve as lookouts for one another—one watching for police and other intruders while the other *cops* (purchases the drugs), prepares the drugs, or injects. Running partners also provide other elements of safety, such as monitoring each other's responses to the drugs they use in order to prevent overdoses or other acute reactions.[73] In this regard, as a 32-year-old former heroin-using prostitute in Miami related in late 1990, for some injection drug users having a running partner can mean the difference between life and death:

Without my partner I'd be dead. He was big, and more than once he saved my ass from being beat on. . . . We weren't lovers or anything like that, although we did sleep together a few times when I was really down. He was no pimp either. We were just really good friends. We could depend on each other.

One time I was cut up pretty bad and he got me patched up. One of my dates [clients] had really worked me over—one of them sado-blood freaks, tied me to a bed and worked over my change purse [vagina] with a coat hanger. Another time when I was bein' ripped off by a bunch of street kids who wanted all of my shit [money and drugs], he came to the rescue, like the fucking Lone Ranger.

For many decades, the sharing of injection equipment has been a prominent aspect of the subculture of the street drug scene, and all of its associated practices are generally learned during initiation to drug use.[74] A user's first episode of sharing is typically unplanned. Since novice injectors rarely have their own *fit* (injection kit or "works"), they often borrow a more experienced user's equipment. After becoming a regular user, association with a running partner may begin and sharing both drugs and needles may serve as a convenience and a symbol of friendship and trust. Since a running partner is often a lover, a surrogate family member, or a replacement family, refusing to share injection equipment could be viewed as an indication of mistrust. For running partners who are also sex partners, injecting drugs as a pair may serve as an even deeper symbol of emotional bonding. In addition, the mixing of blood while injecting and the booting of each other's blood is not uncommon, symbolizing a brotherhood or sisterhood or bond between running partners. For example, as a 22-year old Miami cocaine injector reported in 1993 about herself and her female partner:

Running buddies, yes, and we're also *fuck buddies* and blood sisters. A fuck buddy is when you have sex with someone every so often, with no strings attached. You're not lovers, so you don't care if the person has sex with others. But when you have sex with your buddy you can be yourself, and you do it just to relax. We're blood sisters because every so often when we mix drugs, we boot, and then trade needles. It's a ritual we do now and then. I shoot her drugs and blood and she shoots mine. And it's okay, there's no bone-crusher.*

The risks of such ritual blood exchanges, of course, are obvious, and are likely responsible for HIV and scores of other infections.

Manifestations of HIV Infection Among Injection Drug Users

The clinical spectrum of HIV and AIDS among injection drug users is similar to that of other groups at risk, but with some striking differences in the relative frequency of specific disease manifestations when compared to homosexual men. Injection drug users seem to be at a decreased risk of developing Kaposi's sarcoma,[75] and this was apparent early in the epidemic. Among the first 1,000 cases of AIDS reported in the United States, for example, Kaposi's sarcoma alone was the initial single diagnosis in 36 percent of the 727 homosexual or bisexual men. Another 11 percent had diagnoses of KS and *P. carinii* pneumonia, bringing the total with KS to almost half.[76] By contrast, among the 155 injection drug users in this cohort, only 2.6 percent had KS alone, with an additional 1.3 percent having both KS and *P. carinii*. This striking and significant disease pattern has been consistent, and persists. Yet interestingly, among the homosexual men who were also injection drug users, the incidence of KS was similar to that of non-drug-using homosexuals,[77] suggesting that the link between KS and homosexual practices is more than coincidental.

Differences in occurrence of the opportunistic infections among injection drug users and others at risk have also been noted. The higher frequency of *Pneumocystis carinii* pneumonia among drug injectors compared to homosexual nonusers—68 percent versus 44 percent in New York City—may be due, in part, to the difference in frequency of Kaposi's sarcoma as the initial presenting AIDS diagnosis.[78] Rates of toxoplasmosis, cryptococcosis, and other AIDS-related infections appear to be higher among heterosexual male and female injection drug users than among non-drug-using homosexual men and tend to be intermediate among drug-injecting homosexual men.

These variations in diagnoses among risk groups may be a consequence of differences in previous exposure to infections, or perhaps

---

*When a drug user injects blood of an incompatible type, there is an adverse reaction. Many drug users describe the feeling as similar to having their bones crushed. Hence, a *bone-crusher*.

are related to such demographic factors as geography or socioeconomic status. Alternatively, they may reflect varying modes of acquisition of infectious agents—sexual versus *parenteral* (injected). The increased incidence of pneumonia and other bacterial infections among HIV-infected drug users has been observed in a number of populations. In one small group of injectors hospitalized for conditions other than AIDS—including endocarditis (an infection of the heart valves), pneumonia, and skin infections—the prevalence of HIV seropositivity was 75 percent, whereas among a sample of healthy drug users in a treatment program, 25 percent were seropositive.[79] In addition, there was a correlation between the presence of one of the bacterial infections, HIV seropositivity, and progression to AIDS within four months. The different rates of progression to AIDS in these two populations raised the possibility of an association between common bacterial infections and AIDS.

A higher incidence of HIV "wasting syndrome" has also been noted among injection drug users when compared with others at risk. As noted earlier in the discussion of "slim" disease in Africa, wasting syndrome is a condition involving persistent fever and diarrhea, involuntary weight loss, and chronic weakness.[80] In an analysis of 147,225 AIDS cases reported to the Centers for Disease Control from September 1, 1987, through August 31, 1991, the frequency of wasting syndrome and its association with demographic and risk group variables and with other AIDS-indicator diseases were assessed.[81] A total of 10,525 (7.1 percent) had wasting syndrome as the only AIDS-indicator condition, and 15,726 had wasting syndrome plus at least one other indicator condition. As indicated in Table 3, patients with wasting syndrome as the only AIDS diagnosis were more likely to be female, to be black or Hispanic, and to have a mode of HIV exposure reported as injection drug use, heterosexual contact, or transfusion/hemophilia, with drug injectors representing the largest proportion. Further, as illustrated in Table 4, there were variations by geographic distribution, ranging from 11 percent in the northeastern United States to 47 percent in Puerto Rico. The higher rate among Hispanics was due to the higher prevalence of wasting syndrome in Puerto Rico, which, in turn, was believed to be the result of differences in diagnostic practices and reporting practices, and access to medical care.

Although the reasons for the varied distribution of diseases by AIDS risk behaviors remain uncertain, these differences in the distribution influence the apparent prognosis of HIV infection among intravenous and other injection drug users. The decreased frequency of Kaposi's sarcoma, the increased burden of opportunistic infections and wasting syndrome, and the differences in demography are the most likely explanations for an observed shorter median survival after the diagnosis of AIDS among drug injectors as compared to homosexual men. The median survival time among injection drug users is eight months (some 12 months for homosexual men). However, when homosexual men with Kaposi's sarcoma as the initial AIDS diagnosis are excluded from analysis, the median survival for both male and female injection drug users is similar to that of homosexual men without Kaposi's sarcoma.[82]

Table 3. HIV Wasting Syndrome Among Adult/Adolescent AIDS Patients, United States, 1 September 1987–31 August 1991.

Characteristics	Num-ber	HIV wasting syndrome (%)		HIV wasting syndrome plus Other AIDS Indicator (%)
		No Wasting Syndrome	Wasting Syndrome Only	
Sex				
Male	130852	82.5	6.7	10.7
Female	16373	79.2	10.2	10.6
Race/ethnicity				
White	77811	83.3	5.6	11.1
Black	43384	81.2	7.7	11.1
Hispanic	24447	80.0	11.3	8.8
Asian/other	1503	87.4	3.8	9.2
Exposure category				
Male-to-male sexual contact	83457	84.5	5.0	10.5
IDU	35039	79.3	11.4	9.3
Male-to-male sex plus IDU	9112	77.6	7.8	14.6
Heterosexual contact (IDU)	4955	76.9	9.7	13.4
Heterosexual contact (non-IDU)	3978	79.9	8.0	12.1
Transfusion/hemophilia	4463	74.8	11.2	14.1
Undetermined	6221	84.9	5.1	10.0

Adapted from: Bernard L. Nahlen, Susan Y. Chu, Okey C. Nwanyanwu, Ruth L. Berkelman, Samuel A. Martinez, and John V. Rullan, "HIV Wasting Syndrome in the United States," *AIDS*, 7 (1993), pp. 183-188.

In terms of the natural history of AIDS among injection drug users, the rate of progression of HIV infection to fully expressed AIDS is not available from ongoing prospective natural history studies. Initial impressions indicate that HIV-infected drug injectors progress to clinical disease and AIDS at a rate that may be similar to that of other persons with HIV disease.[83] Furthermore, continuation of drug use behavior may be associated with a worsening of immunologic function and may even be predictive of disease progression.

Throughout the course of their HIV infection, injection drug users present special difficulties in clinical management, primarily due to delays in diagnosing the diseases. Most injectors usually first receive health care related to HIV infection in emergency settings when severe clinical manifestations occur. In the early years of the AIDS epidemic this was partly because members of this subculture perceived their illness as related to drug use rather than HIV infection. However, the more likely continuing reason is their episodic relationships with local health-care systems and a lack of access to ongoing personal health care. Lack of compliance with medical recommendations, health-care workers' disapproval of drug users' lifestyles, poor personal hygiene, and other economic and psychosocial problems also compromise care. Finally, home care and hospice care are often complicated by lack of adequate housing and frequent family disarray.[84]

Table 4. Proportion of AIDS Patients with HIV Wasting Syndrome by Geographic Region and IDU-Associated* Exposure Category, United States, 1 September 1987–31 August 1991

	Number (%) wasting		
Region	**IDU-associated**	**Not IDU-associated**	**All AIDS**
Northeast	23843 (13)	22945 (90)	46788 (11)
North Central	12053 (27)	11136 (19)	23189 (23)
South	12885 (27)	33949 (20)	46834 (22)
West	5571 (22)	28637 (15)	34208 (16)
Puerto Rico	4074 (49)	1452 (1)	5526 (47)

*Includes individuals whose mode of exposure was reported as heterosexual injecting drug users (IDU), male-to-male sexual contact plus IDU, and heterosexual contact with an IDU. Adapted from: Bernard L. Nahlen, Susan Y. Chu, Okey C. Nwanyanwu, Ruth L. Berkelman, Samuel A. Martinez, and John V. Rullan, "HIV Wasting Syndrome in the United States," *AIDS*, 7 (1993), pp. 183–188.

POSTSCRIPT

A backward glance at aspects of the AIDS epidemic reflects a number of curiosities. During July of 1976, amidst the summer-long Bicentennial festivities, a contingent of American Legion war veterans met in Philadelphia to celebrate and reminisce. As they reveled in the spirit of their national birthday, there was a sudden outbreak of fevers, chest congestion, exhaustion, pneumonia, and for some, death.[85] Although the affliction, dubbed "Legionnaire's disease," initially affected only 29 men, it immediately drew the attention of America's mainstream media, all of it—general audience newspapers, news magazines, radio, and network and local television. In 1982, when nine Chicago-area residents died from cyanide-laced Tylenol capsules (followed by a second scare four years later),[86] that event as well received aggressive media coverage. But in 1979, when a New York physician began recognizing a pattern of rare infections among otherwise healthy gay men (and later among injection drug users), it took six years and some 12,000 deaths before the mass media would begin assertive reporting on the phenomena. Perhaps members of the nation's media felt that the deaths of drug addicts and homosexuals just were not worth reporting.

Before long, as the AIDS epidemic spread and HIV became better known, gays and drug injectors came to be looked upon as "carriers" who spread the disease, and others who were infected by them—particularly women and infants—were somehow "innocent victims." Gays and drug injectors were also viewed as members of objectionable populations who had brought the disease upon themselves, through behaviors characteristic of their lifestyles. Beyond that, however, gays and addicts had little else in common.

The striking differences between the two that would significantly affect the course of the AIDS epidemic were the relative sense of "community" that existed in one and not the other, and the ability of gay men to mobilize and become a political force. Most injection drug users were living on the fringes of society—sequestered in shooting galleries, "get-off" houses, and other drug dens, in the streets and alleys and abandoned buildings of America's inner cities, in hospital emergency rooms and drug treatment programs, and in local detention centers and lock-ups as well as state and federal penitentiaries. By contrast, gays were everywhere. They were well represented in the arts, and in every occupation and profession; there were gay physicians and gay social critics, there were gay writers and gay playwrights, and there were gay managers and gay business analysts. There were gay clubs and gay support groups. And perhaps most importantly, there was a gay press.

Although *The Advocate* was founded in Los Angeles in 1967, most of the major gay newspapers began publishing after Stonewall—*Gay Power* in New York at the close of the 1960s, followed by Boston's *Gay Community News*, Washington, D.C.'s *Blade*, *TWIT* in the Southwest, and the *New York Native* during the following decade. Aside from a few papers that concentrated on politics and social commentary, the great majority of the gay papers circulated in neighborhoods where homosexuals congregated—Greenwich Village in New York, for example, or the Castro district in San Francisco—and dealt almost entirely with local community events, with hefty offerings of both sex and humor. When young gay men began dying inexplicably, however, many of the newspapers strayed from the formula.

Gay media involvement in the AIDS epidemic began with a rumor. In mid-May of 1981, while a gay man was visiting his doctor for treatment of a venereal disease, he overheard the physician mention that a number of gays were in intensive care units in New York City for a strange form of pneumonia.[87] Like any good tipster, he called his community newspaper, *New York Native*. At the same time, part-time *Native* reporter Dr. Larry Maas was noticing increasing numbers of mysterious maladies among New York's gay population. Within weeks, Maas's observations became front-page copy in the gay press, and coverage of the new syndrome became significant in the gay community. Also pivotal in this crusade were author/AIDS activist Larry Kramer and journalist Randy Shilts of the *San Francisco Chronicle*. These and other members of the gay journalism fraternity gave a visibility to HIV and AIDS that was unparalleled.

By contrast, there was never such a force in the subculture of drug injectors. Furthermore, there has never been much of a "community" or even a sense of "community" among drug users that could be mobilized for purposes of information dissemination, prevention education, social and emotional support systems, and bonding in the face of crisis. All that drug users had were a few small activist groups and the drug-abuse treatment and research communities. To date, little has changed in this regard.

END NOTES

1. Cited by Dennis Wrong, *Population and Society* (New York: Random House, 1967), p. 100.

2. Cited by Warren Thompson, *Population Problems* (New York: McGraw-Hill, 1953), p. 20.

3. For a discussion of the population debate, see E. P. Hutchinson, *The Population Debate: The Development of Conflicting Theories up to 1900* (New York: Houghton Mifflin, 1967).

4. See Mary Catherine Bateson and Richard Goldsby, *Thinking AIDS: The Social Response to the Biological Threat* (Reading, MA: Addison–Wesley, 1988).

5. For example, see James K. Fitzpatrick, "AIDS: It Is Not Just Another Disease," *The Wanderer,* 15 Aug. 1985, p. 5.

6. Centers for Disease Control, *HIV/AIDS Surveillance*, February 1993.

7. Fintan R. Steele, "A Moving Target: CDC Still Trying to Estimate HIV-1 Seroprevalence," *Journal of NIH Research*, 6 (1994), pp. 25–26.

8. *The Economist*, 22 Nov. 1986, p. 16; *Time*, 1 Dec. 1986, p. 45; *U.S. News & World Report*, 12 Jan. 1987, p. 64; *The New York Times*, 15 Aug. 1987, p. A12.

9. "WorldAIDS Datafile," *WorldAIDS*, May 1993.

10. Jonathan M. Mann, James Chin, Peter Piot, and Thomas Quinn, "The International Epidemiology of AIDS," in Jonathan Piel (ed.), *The Science of AIDS* (New York: W.H. Freeman, 1989), pp. 51–61; Mhairi G. MacDonald and Harold M. Ginzburg, "HIV/AIDS Epidemiology: An Evolving International Pattern," *Pediatric AIDS and HIV Infection: Fetus to Adolescent* 3 (1992), pp. 1–4; J. Chin, P. A. Sato, and J. M. Mann, "Projections of HIV Infections and AIDS Cases to the Year 2000," *Bulletin of the World Health Organization*, 68 (1990), pp. 1–11; Erik Eckholm, "AIDS, Fatally Steady in the U.S., Accelerates Worldwide," *The New York Times*, 28 June 1992, p. E5.

11. See Joseph Feldschuh, *Safe Blood: Purifying the Nation's Blood Supply in the Age of AIDS* (New York: Free Press, 1990).

12. Thomas C. Quinn, "AIDS in Africa: Evidence for Heterosexual Transmission of Human Immunodeficiency Virus," *New York State Journal of Medicine*, 87 (1987), pp. 286–287; *The New York Times*, 24 Nov. 1985, p. 34.

13. *World Press Review*, February 1987, p. 57.

14. Collaborative Study Group of AIDS in Haitian-Americans, "Risk Factors for AIDS Among Haitians Residing in the United States," *Journal of the American Medical Association*, 257 (1987), pp. 636–639.

15. E. Cortes, R. Detels, D. Aboulafia, X. L. Li, T. Moudgil, M. Alam, C. Bonecker, A. Gonzaga, L. Oyafuso, M. Tondo, C. Boite, N. Hammershlak, C. Capitani, D. J. Slamon, and D. D. Ho. "HIV-1, HIV-2, and HTLV-I Infection in High–Risk Groups in Brazil," *New England Journal of Medicine*, 320 (1989), pp. 953–958.

16. See *Time*, 10 Feb. 1990, p. 74; *Newsweek*, 19 Feb. 1990, p. 63; *U.S. News & World Report*, 19 Feb. 1990, pp. 11–12.

17. "Romania's Hidden Epidemic is Revealed," *WorldAIDS*, March 1990, p. 3.

18. Bradley S. Hersh, Florin Popovici, Roxana C. Apertrei, Laurentiu Zolo-tusca, Nicolae Beldescu, Alexandru Calomfirescu, Zdenek Jezek, Margaret J. Oxtoby, Alexander Gromyko, and David L. Haymann, "Acquired Immunodeficiency Syndrome in Romania," *Lancet*, 338 (14 Sept. 1991), pp. 645–649.

19. *The New York Times*, 28 June 1992, p. E5.

20. *The New York Times*, 2 July 1994, p. 8.

21. See Martin Duberman, *Stonewall* (New York: Dutton, 1993).

22. Leigh W. Rutledge, *The Gay Decades* (New York: Plume Books, 1992), p. 2.

23. *The New York Times*, 29 June 1969, p. 33.

24. Rutledge, p. 3.

25. For example, see Todd Gitlin, *The Sixties: Years of Hope, Years of Rage* (New York: Bantam Books, 1987); William Manchester, *The Glory and the Dream: A Narrative History of America, 1932–1972* (Boston: Little, Brown, 1973); Allen J. Matusow, *The Unraveling of America: A History of Liberalism in the 1960s* (New York: Harper & Row, 1984); Charles R. Morris, *A Time of Passion: America, 1960–1980* (New York: Harper & Row, 1984); Milton Viorst, *Fire in the Streets: America in the 1960s* (New York: Simon and Schuster, 1979).

26. Shively's essay, "Indiscriminate Promiscuity as an Act of Revolution," first appeared in a special joint issue of San Francisco's *Gay Sunshine Journal* and Boston's gay liberation paper, *Fag Rag*, published in the Summer of 1974 to commemorate the fifth anniversary of Stonewall. It has been reprinted in Winston Leyland (ed.), *Gay Roots: Twenty Years of Gay Sunshine—An Anthology of Gay History, Sex, Politics, and Culture* (San Francisco: Gay Sunshine Press, 1991), pp. 257–263.

27. John G. Bartlett, Barbara Laughon, and Thomas C. Quinn, "Gastrointestinal Complications of AIDS," in Vincent T. DeVita, Samuel Hellman, and Steven A. Rosenberg (eds.), *AIDS: Etiology, Diagnosis, Treatment, and Prevention* (Philadelphia: Lippincott, 1988), pp. 227–244.

28. B. Frank Polk, Robin Fox, Ron Brookmeyer, Sukon Kanchanaraksa, Richard Kaslow, Barbara Visscher, Charles Rinalso, and John Phair, "Predictors of Acquired Immunodeficiency Syndrome Developing in a Cohort of Seropositive Homosexual Men," *New England Journal of Medicine*, 316 (1987), pp. 61–66.

29. D. M. Auerbach, W. W. Darrow, H. W. Jaffe, and J. W. Curran, "Cluster of Cases of Acquired Immune Deficiency Syndrome: Patients Linked by Sexual Contact," *American Journal of Medicine*, 76 (1984), pp. 487–492.

30. W. Winkelstein, D. M. Lyman, N. Padian, R. Grant, M. Samuel, J. A. Wiley, R. E. Anderson, W. Lang, J. Riggs, and J. A. Levy, "Sexual Practices and Risk of Infection by Human Immunodeficiency Virus: The San Francisco Men's Health Study," *Journal of the American Medical Association*, 257 (1987), pp. 321–325.

31. Warren Winkelstein, Nancy S. Padian, George Rutherford, and Harold F. Jaffe, "Homosexual Men," in Richard A. Kaslow and Donald P. Francis (eds.), *The Epidemiology of AIDS: Expression, Occurrence, and Control of Human Immunodeficiency Virus Type 1 Infection* (New York: Oxford University Press, 1989), pp. 117–135.

32. Winkelstein, Padian, Rutherford, and Jaffe, p. 125.

33. Centers for Disease Control, *HIV/AIDS Surveillance*, 5 (July 1993).

34. See Richard G. Parker, *Bodies, Pleasures and Passions: Sexual Culture in Contemporary Brazil* (Boston: Beacon Press, 1991), pp. 128–129.

35. Winkelstein, Lyman, Padian, et al.

36. Marshall T. Schreeder, Sumner E. Thompson, Stephen C. Hadler, Kenneth R. Berquist, James E. Maynard, David G. Ostrow, Franklyn N. Judson, Irwin Braff, Thomas Nyland, Joseph N. Moore, Pierce Gardner, Irene Doto, and Gladys Reynolds, "Epidemiology of Hepatitis B Infection in Gay Men," *Journal of Homosexuality*, 5 (1980), pp. 307–310.

37. Frank Browning, *The Culture of Desire: Paradox and Perversity in Gay Lives Today* (New York: Crown Publishers, 1993), p. 84.

38. Browning, p. 85–86.

39. Schreeder et al.

40. Mark Nickerson, "Vasodilator Drugs," in Louis S. Goodman and Alfred Gilman (eds.), *The Pharmacological Basis of Therapeutics* (New York: Macmillan, 1975), pp. 727–243.

41. Donald B. Louria, "Sexual Use of Amyl Nitrite," *Medical Aspects of Human Sexuality*, 4 (1970), p. 89; Richard Seymour and David E. Smith, *Guide to Psychoactive Drugs* (New York: Harrington Park Press, 1987), p. 40.

42. Harry W. Haverkos, "Nitrite Inhalants: History, Epidemiology, and Possible Links to AIDS," under review.

43. Institute of Medicine, National Academy of Sciences, *Mobilizing Against AIDS* (Cambridge: National Academy Press, 1989), p. 94.

44. Guy R. Newell, Peter W. A. Mansell, Margaret R. Spitz, James M. Reuben, and Evan M. Hersh, "Volatile Nitrites: Use and Adverse Effects Related to the Current Epidemic of the Acquired Immune Deficiency Syndrome," *American Journal of Medicine*, 78 (1985), pp. 811–816; Robert Root-Bernstein, *Rethinking AIDS: The Tragic Cost of Premature Consensus* (New York: Free Press, 1993), p. 126.

45. Harry W. Haverkos, "Nitrite Inhalant Abuse and AIDS-Related Kaposi's Sarcoma," *Journal of Acquired Immune Deficiency Syndromes*, 3, Supp 1 (1990), pp. S47–S50.

46. Enoch Gordis, "Alcohol and AIDS," National Institute on Alcohol Abuse and Alcoholism, *Alcohol Alert*, 15 (January 1992).

47. See James A. Inciardi, *The War on Drugs II: The Continuing Epic of Heroin, Cocaine, Crack, Crime, AIDS, and Public Policy* (Mountain View, CA: Mayfield, 1992), pp. 93–94.

48. John L. Martin, "Drug Use and Unprotected Anal Intercourse Among Gay Men," *Health Psychology*, 9 (1990), pp. 450–465.

49. See Charles Silverstein and Felice Picano, *The New Joy of Gay Sex* (New York: Harper/Collins, 1992), pp. 156–157.

50. Thomas C. Quinn and King K. Holmes, "Proctitis Proctocolitis, and Enteritis in Homosexual Men," in King K. Holmes, Per-Anders Mardh, P. Frederick Sparling, and Paul J. Wiesner (eds.), *Sexually Transmitted Diseases* (New York: McGraw-Hill, 1984), pp. 672–691.

51. Root-Bernstein, p. 227.

52. N. Sohn and J. G. Robilotti, "The Gay Bowel Syndrome: A Review of Colonic and Rectal Conditions in 200 Male Homosexuals," *American Journal of Gastroenterology*, 67 (1977), p. 478.

53. H. Most, "Manhattan: A Tropical Isle?" *American Journal of Tropical Medicine and Hygiene*, 17 (1968), pp. 333–354.

54. R. B. Pearce, "Intestinal Protozoal Infections and AIDS," *Lancet*, 2 (1983), p. 51.

55. Donald I. Abrams, "The Relationship Between Kaposi's Sarcoma and Intestinal Parasites Among Homosexual Males in the United States," *Journal of Acquired Immune Deficiency Syndromes*, 3, Supp. 1 (1990), pp. S44–S46.

56. Winkelstein, Padian, Rutherford, and Jaffe.

57. Institute of Medicine, National Academy of Sciences, *Confronting AIDS: Directions for Public Health, Health Care, and Research* (Washington, DC: National Academy Press, 1986), p. 45.

58. D. A. Cooper, P. Maclean, and R. Finlayson, *Lancet*, 1 (1985), pp. 537–540; R. Fox, L. J. Eldred, E. J. Fuchs, *AIDS* 1 (1987), p. 35; R. Goldman, W. Lang, D. Lyman, *American Journal of Medicine*, 18 (1986), p. 1122.

59. Winkelstein, Padian, Rutherford, and Jaffe, p. 129.

60. Winkelstein, Padian, Rutherford, and Jaffe, p. 129.

61. Winkelstein, Padian, Rutherford, and Jaffe, p. 130.

62. Steven Petrow, *Dancing Against the Darkness: A Journey Through America in the Age of AIDS* (Lexington, MA: Lexington Books, 1990), pp. 166–167.

63. Dale D. Chitwood, James A. Inciardi, Duane C. McBride, Clyde B. McCoy, H. Virginia McCoy, and Edward Trapido, *A Community Approach to AIDS Intervention: Exploring the Miami Outreach Project for Injecting Drug Users and Other High Risk Groups* (Westport, CT: Greenwood Press, 1991), pp. 89–90.

64. John Kaplan, *The Hardest Drug: Heroin and Public Policy* (Chicago: University of Chicago Press, 1983), p. 10; Michael M. Baden, "Methadone Related Deaths in New York City," *International Journal of the Addictions*, 5 (1975), pp. 489–498.

65. James A. Inciardi, "AIDS—A Strange Disease of Uncertain Origins," *American Behavioral Scientist*, 33 (1990), pp. 397–407.

66. L. K. Resnick, S. Z. Veren, S. Salahuddin, S. Tondreau, and P. D. Karkham, "Stability and Inactivation of HTLV-III/LAV Under Clinical and Laboratory Environments," *Journal of the American Medical Association*, 255 (1986), pp. 1887–1891.

67. F. T. Barre-Sinoussi, M. T. Nugeyre, and J. C. Chermann, "Resistance of AIDS Virus at Room Temperature," *Lancet* (28 Sept.), pp. 721–722; L. S. Martin, J. S. McDougal, and S. L. Lsokoski, "Disinfection and Inactivation of the Human T Lymphotropic Virus Type III/ Lymphadenopathy-Associated Virus," *Journal of Infectious Diseases*, 152 (1985), pp. 400–403.

68. Paul Shapshak, Clyde B. McCoy, Syed M. Shah, J. Bryan Page, James E. Rivers, Norman L. Weatherby, Dale D. Chitwood, and Deborah C. Mash, "Preliminary Laboratory Studies of Inactivation of HIV-1 in Needles and Syringes Containing Infected Blood Using Undiluted Household Bleach," *Journal of Acquired Immune Deficiency Syndromes*, 7 (1994), pp. 754–759.

69. S. Koester, R. Booth, and W. Wiebel, "The Risk of HIV Transmission from Sharing Water, Drug Mixing Containers and Cotton Filters Among Intravenous Drug Users," *International Journal on Drug Policy* 1 (1990), pp. 28–30.

70. Koester, Booth, and Wiebel; J. P. C. Grund, C. D. Kaplan, and N. F. P. Adriaans, "Needle Exchange and Drug Sharing: A View from Rotterdam." *Newsletter of the International Working Group on AIDS and IV Drug Use,* 4 (1989), pp. 4–5; J. P. C. Grund, C. D. Kaplan, N. F. P. Adriaans, P. Blanken, and J. Huisman, "The Limitations of the Concept of Needle Sharing: The Practice of Frontloading," *AIDS,* 4 (1990), pp. 819–821.

71. James A. Inciardi and J. Bryan Page, "Drug Sharing Among Intravenous Drug Users," *AIDS,* 5 (1991), pp. 772–774.

72. James A. Inciardi, Dorothy Lockwood, and Judith A. Quinlan, "Drug Use in Prison: Patterns, Processes, and Implications for Treatment," *Journal of Drug Issues,* 23 (1993), pp. 119–129.

73. Don C. Des Jarlais, Samuel R. Friedman, and David Strug, "AIDS and Needle Sharing Within the IV–Drug Use Subculture," in Douglas A. Feldman and Thomas M. Johnson (eds.), *The Social Dimensions of AIDS: Methods and Theory* (New York: Praeger, 1986), pp. 111–126.

74. John A. O'Donnell and J. P. Jones, "Diffusion of the Intravenous Technique Among Narcotic Addicts," *Journal of Health and Social Behavior* 9 (1968), pp. 120–130; Richard C. Stephens and Duane C. McBride, "Becoming a Street Addict," *Human Organization,* 15 (1976), pp. 87–93.

75. Kenneth B. Hymes, "Kaposi's Sarcoma and AIDS," in Gary P. Wormser, Rosalyn E. Stahl, and Edward J. Bottone (eds.), *AIDS and Other Manifestations of HIV Infection* (Park Ridge, NJ: Noyes Publications, 1987), pp. 747–766; Paul A. Volberding, "Kaposi's Sarcoma in AIDS," in Jay A. Levy (ed.), *AIDS: Pathogenesis and Treatment* (New York: Marcel Dekker, 1989), pp. 345–358.

76. Gerald Friedland, "Parenteral Drug Users," in Kaslow and Francis, pp. 153–178.

77. Friedland, p. 166.

78. Don C. Des Jarlais, Eric Wish, Samuel R. Friedman, Rand Stoneburner, Stanley R. Yancovitz, Donna Mildvan, Waffa El-Sadr, Elizabeth Brady, and Mary Cuadrado, "Intravenous Drug Use and the Heterosexual Transmission of the Human Immunodeficiency Virus: Current Trends in New York City," *New York State Journal of Medicine,* 87 (1987), pp. 283–286; New York City Department of Health, "The AIDS Epidemic in New York City, 1981–1984: New York City Department of Health AIDS Surveillance," *American Journal of Epidemiology,* 123 (1986), pp. 1013–1025.

79. Daniel Shine, Bernice Moll, Eugene Emeson, Ilya Spigland, Carol Harris, Catherine Butkus Small, Gerald Friedland, Stanley H. Weiss, and Anne J. Bodner, "Serologic, Immunologic, and Clinical Features of Parenteral Drug Users from Contrasting Populations," *American Journal of Drug and Alcohol Abuse,* 13 (1987), pp. 401–412.

80. Institute of Medicine, National Academy of Sciences, *Mobilizing Against AIDS* (Washington, DC: National Academy Press, 1989), p. 62.

81. Bernard L. Nahlen, Susan Y. Chu, Okey C. Nwanyanwu, Ruth L. Berkelman, Samuel A. Martinez, and John V. Rullan, "HIV Wasting Syndrome in the United States," *AIDS,* 7 (1993), pp. 183–188.

82. Brian R. Saltzman, Mary R. Motyl, Gerald H. Friedland, John C. McKitrick, and Robert S. Klein, "Mycobacterium Tuberculosis Bacteremia in the Acquired Immunodeficiency Syndrome," *Journal of the American Medical Association*, 256 (1986), pp. 390–391; New York City Department of Health.

83. Des Jarlais et al. 1987.

84. Wilma Bulkin, Lucille Brown, Deborah Fraioli, Emily Giannattasio, Gerilyn McGuire, Patrice Tyler, and Gerald Friedland, "Hospice Care of the Intravenous Drug User AIDS Patient in a Skilled Nurse Facility," *Journal of Acquired Immune Deficiency Syndromes*, 1 (1988), pp. 375–80.

85. Peter N. Carroll, *It Seemed Like Nothing Happened: The Tragedy and Promise of America in the 1970s* (New York: Holt, Rinehart, and Winston, 1982), p. 306.

86. *Time* 24 Feb. 1986, p. 22; *Newsweek*, 26 Feb. 1986, p. 25.

87. Kinsella, p. 25.

CHAPTER THREE

Bathhouses, Shooting Galleries, and Other Reservoirs of Infection

Two characteristic features of the American drug scene have been the variety of subcultures in which alternative patterns of substance use have been concentrated and the numerous different habitats in which certain forms of alcohol use and drug-taking repeatedly occur. Perhaps best known in this regard was the "speak" or "speakeasy," the illicit liquor shop of the Prohibition Era. There were numerous types of speakeasies, each with its own clientele. At the bottom of the scale in the big cities were the "clip joints," "cab joints," or "steer joints" that preyed on unwary locals or visitors unfamiliar with city life. The alcohol was always on hand, and so were the women who worked in the sex industry, but the prices for both were always outrageously high.[1] At the other end of the spectrum were the more "uptown" establishments, often found in brownstone residences and operating under the guise of "clubs." These locations catered to the more fashionable and "well-to-do" urbanites.[2]

Outside the cities and somewhat lesser known in American folklore were the "roadhouses." Even before Prohibition, some city and town neighborhoods had closed their saloons, but the operations quickly relocated beyond the village corporate limits. In states and counties that had elected to be "dry," a similar situation evolved. Given many persons' attitudes toward drinking, brawling, loud music, and women in tight dresses, such "indecencies" could not be tolerated as they might have been in the larger cities. For those who wished to drink, roadhouses became country traditions. The liquor flowed freely and the jukeboxes were loud, but the lights were typically low enough so that no one would be recognized.[3] As was the case in many of the "speaks," "bar girls" were available for a price.

Also well-known were the opium dens that existed from the mid-nineteenth through the early twentieth century in San Francisco and New York. They were places for smoking, as well as meeting places for members of the underworlds of vice and crime to gather in relative safety to enjoy a smoke (of opium, hashish, or tobacco) with friends and associates. For the addict, they were places to find opium, opium-smoking paraphernalia, and the company of other opium smokers. In a sense, these establishments were a social institution.[4] More "respectable" but short-lived counterparts of the opium den were the "hashish clubs" of the 1880s. Catering to a clientele of writers, artists, and other members of the *avant garde*, they could be found on the back streets of almost every major city from New York to San Francisco.[5]

In addition to drinking alcohol and/or using drugs, people have typically congregated in a variety of different establishments for the purpose of sexual activity. Prostitution was a common feature in many speakeasies and roadhouses, and history has for centuries documented the existence of houses of prostitution.[6] The modern counterparts of the opium dens, speaks, and brothels are the gay bathhouses and sex clubs that emerged in the 1970s, the shooting galleries and "get-off" houses associated with injection drug use, and the crack joints and other drug dens of late twentieth-century America. Of significance here are the roles they play in the transmission of HIV and AIDS.

ASPECTS OF THE GAY SEX SCENE

Playwright, novelist, and polemicist Larry Kramer is considered one of the nation's leading AIDS activists. HIV-positive since 1988 and recently described by *Playboy* magazine as "a master of ad hominem invective,"[7] Kramer has been considered controversial. He once called Dr. Anthony Fauci, head of the National Institute of Health's AIDS effort, a "murderer"; he labeled actress Elizabeth Taylor a "dilettante"; and remarked that fashion designer Calvin Klein was "married to his dick." On the Reagan/Bush AIDS effort he emphatically stated:

> The door to the White House was cemented shut on anything that remotely went against their agenda. Talking to them was like howling in the wind. We could have had people by the hundreds setting fire to themselves in front of the White House and it would not have made the slightest bit of difference. They were simply not going to pay any attention. Reagan was out to lunch, and the person who was in charge of AIDS under Reagan was a horror show called Gary Bauer. He was just a beady-eyed shit. He is still a hateful man who loathes every homosexual who ever walked the earth. He was going to see to it that we couldn't get anywhere near the White House. And the same held true for John Sununu and the Bush playhouse.[8]

Born in 1935 in Bridgeport, Connecticut, Kramer remembered his childhood as particularly miserable. He hated sports, and his father considered him a sissy. By the time he was 12 he knew that he was "different," and during his first year at Yale, lonely and isolated, he attempted suicide by swallowing some 200 aspirins. It was then that he first admitted to anyone that he was gay. After he finished college, Kramer's literary talents began to flourish. By the early 1960s, he was a producing executive at Columbia Pictures, and in 1970 he won an Oscar nomination for his screenplay in the United Artist production of "Women in Love." In 1977, just prior to the beginning of the AIDS crisis, his first novel, *Faggots*[9], was published. Less than four years later, on a summer evening in 1981 while visiting a dying friend on New York's Fire Island, Kramer had his first glimpse at what would become known as AIDS. A month later he helped form Gay Men's Health Crisis, the first grass-roots organization in the United States to combat the AIDS epidemic. Kramer is also the founder of ACT UP—the AIDS Coalition to Unleash Power—an international army of AIDS activists.

Kramer's *Faggots*, perhaps the most controversial piece of gay literature to appear in recent memory, brought him mixed visibility in the gay community. A graphically sexual novel chronicling gay life in America, it was the saga of 39-year-old Fred Lemish and his longing and looking for a man for permanence, commitment, and love. But Fred seemed always to be looking for Mr. Right in the wrong places, from New York's downtown Everhard Baths, to the Pines of Fire Island, to the mythical "pits" and "meat racks" where all manner of male flesh might be found.

Kramer, with his comment that "Of the 2,639,857 faggots in the New York City area, 2,639,857 think primarily with their cocks,"[10] had intended *Faggots* to be a parody. And in many ways it was, but it was also criticized by parts of the gay community and reviled in segments of straight America. In 1989, Kramer recalled:

> I thought I'd written a satirical novel about the gay life I and most of my friends were living. I'd meant it to be funny. Even though the book was a best seller . . . I found myself actually shunned by friends.[11]

In terms of *why* so many in gay America criticized the book, the problem was what appeared to be the theme of sexual sin. University of Western Ontario arts professor James Miller offered the following perspective on *Faggots*:

> What made Kramer's novel so controversial, at least in New York, was not its thunderous revelation that Fire Island was really hell . . . but rather his Old Testament moralizations on fucking the trash on the beach and fisting the meat on the rack. Consciences were pricked. Pricks were exposed to the anaphrodisiac strokes of conscience. . . . No televangelist in the service of the Heterosexist panopticon could have

poured a colder shower on the boys in the sand than an informed source like Kramer—a dancer from their own dance. Much to their embarrassed surprise, he was utterly serious in his condemnation of their "Beatific Vision" as a glamorous illusion, a trashing of the high ideals of Gay Culture in a Gehenna [the biblical "valley of slaughter"] of lost souls.[12]

For much of straight America, *Faggots* graphically described what were considered by many to be the less appealing aspects of the gay scene—the fisting, *felching* ("fuck my friend and I'll suck your come out of his asshole"),[13] and orgies involving numerous, anonymous partners of the same sex. Perhaps most strikingly, *Faggots* was the first best-selling novel to describe the gay baths to a homophobic mainstream America.

The Gay Baths

They went by many names—baths, bathhouses, steam baths, Turkish baths, and the like, and the best-known and most popular were the Mine Shaft, Everhard, Continental, and St. Marks Baths in New York; and in San Francisco, the Hothouse, Bulldog (which celebrated its third anniversary on October 11, 1981 with a "Biggest Cock in S.F." contest), and Castro Steam Baths. Nominally, they were places with lounges, steam rooms, and saunas for people to relax and meet with friends, but journalist Randy Shilts commented otherwise in the *New York Native* in 1984, well into the AIDS epidemic:

> By the mid 1970s promiscuity was less a lifestyle than an article of faith. Before long an entire subculture and business network emerged catering to drugged-out alcoholic gay men with penchants for kinky promiscuous sexual acts. And so in cities across America bathhouses opened their doors, unprecedented in that they were businesses created solely for the purpose of quick multiple sex acts, often accomplished without so much as a word.[14]

The many hundreds of gay baths that thrived in San Francisco, New York, Boston, and other urban centers all seemed to share a number of characteristics.[15] Significant features included mazes of dimly lighted passageways, dark stairways, and red lights. Almost everywhere men could be seen—some naked, but most in the traditional bathhouse suit—a towel, occasionally with a safety pin in the corner. And there were endless variations on the towel wrap: long and tight like a Polynesian sarong; loose, disheveled, and barely hanging on in *Odd Couple* fashion; folded once like a taut mini, or twice for a sumo skirt; or perhaps in a type of culotte adaptation, open in front like a curtain in a display case.

Most bathhouses had one or more lounges—darkened rooms with wall-to-wall cushioned benches, and perhaps a table in the center with

AIDS literature arrayed. The atmosphere of the lounges was one of both lethargy and anticipation—the lethargy of the postcoital state along with the communicating glances and brushings, the silent bargainings in advance of expected and hoped-for sexual encounters. Most of the baths also had steam rooms, saunas, and Jacuzzis where the same types of scenes could be observed, perhaps even of men having sex.

All bathhouses had dark rooms and cramped corridors leading to the cubicles where many of the sexual activities occurred. The cubicles were small, each just large enough to accommodate a mattress or raised pallet. Characteristic as well were the wooden dividers separating one cubicle from the next, stopping well below the ceiling. Although each cubicle had a door with a number clearly marked, the doors were often left open. In any given cubicle one might observe a man lying on his back, naked or decorated with a towel, eyeing the doorway, waiting for someone to enter. Elsewhere, either in a cubicle or a passageway, a man might be sitting or walking past with his erection in his hands. Down the hallway or in the next cubicle two men might be embracing, engaging in oral or anal sex, masturbating, or silently resting after having had sex.

Characteristic of *all* of the gay baths was a commercialization of frequent, anonymous, high-risk sexual activity in which epidemics of venereal disease, hepatitis, and enteric disorders thrived. And it is not surprising that with regard to HIV and AIDS, the baths were considered frequent sources of infection by public-health authorities. Furthermore, beginning in the spring of 1983, at the peak of AIDS coverage in the national media, closing the baths became a heated issue in New York, San Francisco, and elsewhere. The debate concerned a municipality's responsibilities for public health versus the right of individuals to control their own lifestyles.[16] In the end, public-health concerns prevailed and bathhouses were closed in many jurisdictions, and were tightly controlled in others. Although most of the bathhouses had been closed by the late 1980s, within a year or two others began to reopen. Visits to gay baths in New York, Miami, and Los Angeles suggest that little may have changed.

The following observations were made by one of the authors as part of a 1993 ethnographic study of six bathhouses and sex clubs. Although each location had its own unique features, a composite of their general characteristics is presented here.

> After paying a fee and entering, an attendant wordlessly hands you a basket for your possessions and a key to a locker. You move immediately to a locker room, similar to those at the YMCA, only this one has several full-length mirrors and one or two condom dispensers. With a towel wrapped around your middle, in whatever fashion best fits your personality and/or physical stature, you pass to the next room. It may be a lounge or T.V. room in which a pornographic movie plays silently. In

either case, there are several toweled men—some in couples, touching, a few talking, others sitting alone, watching and waiting. As you enter the room, many eyes look your way—some lingering, hoping for a sign of interest or acquiescence, while others immediately turn away.

In the dim corridors, nude figures of every shape and size seem to prowl. Naked men stand in doorways to cubicles, some with erections, many touching themselves, a few slowly masturbating, and almost all making eye contact. As you pass, there is some physical contact—delicate brushings on the back, chest, or rear from one side, while someone on the other side may gently cup your testicles and then your penis, unless you push his hand away. In the cubicles, with doors left open and signs that read "one occupant only," naked bodies lie on cots. Occasionally, a man will enter and the door will close. There are periodic moans, and a faint scent of marijuana fills the air. For some the doors never close. Sexual embraces, oral, and anal sex are in view of passersby. Sometimes a third party may enter to join a couple, to watch, or to be sent away.

There is a larger room, also dimly lighted, where a sea of twisting flesh keeps changing shape. As one man fondles another, a bystander guides his neighbor's penis into the rectum of a third party. The scene changes again, shifting intermittently from random couplings to daisy chains of oral sex. Then suddenly, as three men enter the room, all contacts are broken and movement ceases. There is an air of excitement and anticipation, as if something momentous is about to happen, something that the revelers have been waiting for—the "main event," so to speak. All eyes are transfixed on the three, all perfectly sculptured men, slim but well-muscled, handsome and young, and all have large, erect penises. At first they are frolicsome—touching, caressing, kissing. After a few minutes, however, they seem to be ready for something. One of the men, dark-haired and the largest of the three, lies down facing most of the onlookers, with his back on the floor. The second, light-haired but with a thick black mustache, moves to his knees and straddles the dark-haired man, face-to-face. Leaning slightly forward, he becomes the receptive partner, as the man on the floor arches his body and slowly eases his penis into his first partner's rectum. As the two men engage in a sensuous, slow-motion rendering of anal intercourse, the third man, a blond, watches from behind, fondling his own erection. After a time, the light-haired man, the receptive partner, eases further forward with his hands outstretched on either side of the other man's head, touching the floor to support his weight. The faces of the two are only centimeters apart. The blond then moves forward, removes the dark-haired man's penis from the rectum of the other, clasps it tightly to his own, and then gently but firmly and swiftly inserts the two organs into the anus of the kneeling man. As the spectacle continues, watchers come and go, back to the cubicles or to the showers or sauna where other connections might be made. Others remain, wondering if the trio will be inviting others to join them.

In the midst of the activity, safe sex messages are not inconspicuous. Over the door of one room a sign reads, "USE A CONDOM, OR BEAT IT!" On the opposite wall, a poster containing a faded picture of Rock Hudson carries the message, "DON'T BECOME A STATISTIC, PRACTICE SAFE SEX, USE A CONDOM." Even in the presence of numerous vending machines containing any variety and hue of condoms, few seem to be in use.

The 1990s Gay Sex Clubs

The reappearance of the gay baths in the late 1980s and early 1990s was part of a wider proliferation of commercial sex establishments that occurred in most major cities. Now known as "sex clubs," they range from bathhouses and bars to movie houses and bookstores where patrons pay an entrance fee to have sex in open areas or closed rooms.[17] Some are little more than designated rooms in bars, theaters, and bookstores, and several cater to both gay and straight customers. In pornographic bookstores, there may be private video rooms large enough for two. In others, the viewing booths may have "glory holes," which are fist-sized openings to an adjoining booth, 30 inches off the floor—just large enough to accommodate a hand or penis. Booths in slightly better establishments have benches and a tissue or paper towel dispenser anchored to the wall.

There are many reasons for the advent and growth of the new sex clubs. First, there seems to be a generation gap in AIDS awareness. Fewer of the younger gay men have seen friends and lovers die of AIDS; accordingly, they are more likely than their elders to have multiple partners and practice unprotected intercourse. Second, many young gays carry a conviction of indestructibility along with the belief that AIDS happens only to older men. As a 22-year-old college senior from Syracuse, New York, recently commented:

> Personally, I've never met anyone with AIDS. I just don't know anybody who's got it. From what I can see it's the older group, the thirty-somethings and forty-pluses that hang out in the New York and San Francisco leather bars.

Third, there is a significant knowledge gap between old and young. Few schools provide intensive AIDS prevention programs, and virtually none broaches such taboo subjects as homosexuality and gay sex. It is for this reason that AIDS prevention workers hear such statements as:

> I know I can't get AIDS so long as I have sex just with my own age group, so long as they are healthy, I keep myself clean and make sure I get tested, and pull out before I come.

Moreover, many education programs fail to teach youths—straight or gay—to negotiate condom use effectively. Many young gay men fear that if they even suggest using a condom they will be suspected of being HIV-positive.

Fourth, there are many gay men of all ages who are fatalistic about AIDS. A 40-year-old Miami man commented in 1993:

> I've seen lots of my friends die from AIDS, and they were practicing safe sex most of the time. No matter what, we're all going to get it.

Many of these same men, furthermore, are beginning to tire of condom use. Or as the Miami man quoted above stated: "I'm sick of screwing a piece of latex."

Several cities have made a concerted effort to make the new sex clubs safer. In New York, clubs are now required to distribute condoms, provide adequate lighting, and train monitors to supervise sexual activity; in Los Angeles and other locales, clubs must restrict sexual activity and submit to regular government inspections.[18] And of growing popularity are the so-called "J.O." (jack-off) clubs, an outgrowth of organized parties by gay men who practice masturbation.[19] What makes J.O. clubs different is that oral and anal penetration are forbidden. Rather than lying around on beds, cots, or couches, most men stand, in various stages of undress, moving from one group to another, with hand towels and lubricants readily available. However, even in the well-intentioned and best-policed clubs, unsafe sex often happens and HIV and other sexually transmitted diseases are regular, however uninvited, guests.

SHOOTING GALLERIES AND INJECTION DRUG USE

The bathhouses represent potential reservoirs of infection for gay and bisexual men. For injection drug users and their sex partners, *shooting galleries* may be considered to share the same appellation. In most urban locales where rates of injection drug use are high, common sites for injecting drugs (and sometimes for purchasing drugs) are the neighborhood "shooting galleries," typically referred to in some settings as *safe houses*, and in Miami as *get-off houses*. After purchasing heroin, cocaine, amphetamines, or some other injectable substance in a local *copping* (drug selling) area, users are faced with three logistical problems: how to get off the street quickly to avoid arrest for possession of drugs, where to obtain a set of *works* (drug paraphernalia) with which to administer the drugs, and where to find a safe place to *get off* (inject the drugs). As such, shooting galleries occupy a functional niche in the world of injection drug use, where for a fee of two or three dollars users can rent an injection kit and relax while "getting off." After using a syringe and needle, the user generally returns them to a central storage place in the gallery where they are held until someone else rents them. On many occasions, however, these "works" are simply passed to another user in the gallery.

Gallery Characteristics and Roles

In Miami and elsewhere, shooting galleries have not been systematically studied. However, based on the investigators' observations combined with reports from a variety of ethnographic and other research studies in drug communities in several parts of the United States,[20] their more obvious roles and characteristics can be described. Most shooting galleries are situated in basements and backrooms, apartments and hotel rooms, and even in house trailers in the rundown sections of cities where drug use rates are high. Typically, they are only sparsely furnished, and cleanliness is absent. Reports suggest many similarities from city to city. In West Oakland, California, for example:

> [The gallery was] in a ratty, condemned house up over an old-time nightclub. They used two rooms and a hallway. It had lights, but no running water, and they just shit out the windows. And the lights were hooked up from outside, you know, somebody else's shit.[21]

And in Miami, an outreach worker described a popular get-off house as follows:

> The place is really gross. It's just a small house with an upstairs, in the middle of the block set further back than the other houses and has a garage in the back. The owner lives upstairs and uses part of the downstairs. There are two back rooms which he uses as the get-off and they're cut off from his front rooms by wood paneling nailed over the doorway. It's filthy, probably not ever been cleaned.

> There's an old couch, two tables, couple of chairs, some buckets. One room is real small, and has a sink that works—probably was a kitchen at one time. No bathroom, so they piss in the sink, or right on the floor or out the windows. Smells like it too. One of the windows has no glass, so sometimes there's all kinds of creepies to watch out for. There's all kinds of junk on the floors, like needle wrappers, old needles and syringes that don't work any more, bloody cotton and band-aids. Stuff like that. In the corner of the room there's a table with three or four containers of syringes. They look like the Chinese food take-out buckets. There's matches on the table, and a file to sharpen needles, some caps and baby food jars for water, and a bag of cotton balls.

Other galleries are in abandoned buildings, darkened hallways, alleys, and under railroad bridges and highway ramps. Characterized by the stench of urine and littered with trash, human feces, garbage, and discarded injection paraphernalia, the conditions are extremely unsanitary. Rarely is there heat, running water, or functional plumbing. For example, an informant in Miami reported:

Before the county came along and cleaned out the junkies and the homeless, there was this section under Route 395 near Biscayne Boulevard known as the "shit hole." There were some dumpsters up at one end near the walls of the overpass. When you were behind them you could see out but no one could see you, so there would be folks shooting up back there on and off every day and night.

Most galleries are run by drug users, drug dealers, and drug user/dealers. Neighborhood heroin and/or cocaine sellers may operate galleries as a service to customers—providing users with a nearby location to inject for a slight charge, perhaps two or three dollars. More often, however, gallery operators are drug users themselves who provide a service for a small fee or a *taste* (sample) of someone else's drugs.

For the majority of injection drug users, shooting galleries are considered the least desirable places to patronize. Most prefer to use their own homes or apartments or those of drug-using friends. These are considered safer than galleries, and there are few users who relish having to pay a fee to use someone else's drug paraphernalia. For a minority of hard-core injectors, there is also the matter of personal hygiene. As one heroin user summed it up:

> Galleries ain't where it's at. We wasn't brought up like that. They be definitely hardcore junkies and they don't give a damn no more about how their appearance is or nothing like that. Ain't nobody want to give another two dollars. Their works . . . all dirty, man. An' people be shootin' blood all over you.[22]

For many drug injectors, however, the use of shooting galleries is routine and commonplace. Moreover, there are repeated occasions in the lives of all injection drug users, including the most hygienically fastidious types, when galleries become necessary. If they have no works of their own, or if friends or other running partners have no works, then a neighborhood gallery is the only recourse. Similarly, users who purchase drugs far from home also gravitate toward the galleries. This tendency is based on the heightened risk of arrest when one carries drugs and drug paraphernalia over long stretches. In addition, for the heroin or cocaine user undergoing withdrawal, getting somewhere close by to inject after copping is imperative. Moreover, the gallery operator often serves as a middleman between drug user and drug dealer, thus making the get-off house the locus of exchange. For example, as one Miami heroin user explained the situation 1988:

> Okay, let's say I'm white, but the only place I can cop some smack [heroin] is in the black neighborhoods, but I'm afraid that I'll be ripped off [robbed] there. But, then there's this gallery an' I know the man there, he's right [trusted] by the buyers and sellers. So I go there an' he cops for me for a few dollars and maybe a taste. For another $3 I can use his works and house to lay up in for a little while.

Finally, there are drug injectors who actually prefer local galleries because of the opportunities they provide to socialize with other drug users. For example, a Miami cocaine user explained in 1993:

> When you live on the street you need a place to go, to see people, to relax, to hear things, to be in the know. You need to connect with your friends, with your running partners; you need to know where the drugs are, where the police are working, who the snitches are, where the fences are, who's in jail and who's out, who's HIV positive and who's bought it with an OD [overdosed], and who's full of shit and who isn't.

Interestingly, this clearinghouse role is not something unique to shooting galleries and the drug scene. Criminal "hangouts" have served the identical role for a variety of segments of the underworld down through the ages. For example, a Brooklyn-born sneak thief and burglar with a criminal history spanning the Prohibition Era through the late 1960s once reflected on some of New York City's hangouts for professional thieves:

> The bars along 48th and 49th Streets from 6th to 8th Avenues are to me what the golf and country clubs are to the execs. That's where we do *our* business, where we meet key people, and where we relax. Whenever you get in town you know where you need to go and each of us has our favorites.[23]

There are other reasons for using a shooting gallery. For homeless persons, there is nowhere else to go. For those with no money or drugs, hanging out in a gallery is a way to get some free drugs—a taste at any rate. Also, the gallery is a place where the user can find a *street doc* or *house doc*. More specifically, some users are squeamish about sticking needles into their veins and injecting themselves. Some are just not particularly adept at it. Others, because of deep or collapsed veins, cannot orchestrate a proper *hit* or *register* (drops of blood in the syringe as evidence of connecting with the vein).[24] Under these circumstances, the street or house "doc" will inject the drugs into the user for a small fee (money or a "taste" of drugs). For example, a heroin and cocaine-using house doc in Miami reported in 1992:

> I was a med-tech in Nam, so I've had a lot of experience. I can shoot into any vein in the body—arms, legs, neck, between the fingers and toes, wherever. Most of the time I just sit here and wait 'till someone comes in and wants me to fix them. Sometimes I got to make house calls, to an apartment, a house, an alley, a car. Someone comes and tells me, and I go make the call. That's why they call me the "doc." And some docs simply sell their skills and rely on house works, but I carry my own outfit. I keep it clean, and people know that, so they always call me.

In short, despite its lack of hygiene, the shooting gallery does indeed occupy a functional role in the street worlds of injection drug-taking and drug-seeking.

Shooting Galleries and HIV

As mentioned briefly in Chapter Two, the sharing of hypodermic needles, syringes, and other parts of the injection kit is the most likely route of HIV acquisition and transmission among injection drug users. The mechanism is the exchange of the blood of the previous user that is lodged in the needle, the syringe, or elsewhere. Because most injection drug use is intravenous (into a vein), the very nature of "mainlining" is such that contact between the paraphernalia and the user's blood is virtually guaranteed. The transmission problem is exacerbated through the practice of *booting*, also known as *kicking*. As noted previously, booting involves the use of a syringe to draw blood from the user's arm, the mixing of the drawn blood with the drug already taken into the syringe, and the injection of the blood/drug mixture into the vein.

There are three reasons for booting. First, most injectors draw blood into the syringe for the sake of "vein registration," that is, to insure that the needle is properly placed in the vein. Second, many injectors draw large amounts of blood into the syringe, pumping it in and out several times to mix the blood with the drug solution. Users believe that this practice potentiates a drug's effects. Third, many users wish to test the strength or effect of the drug before injecting the entire amount.[25] In any case, booting leaves traces of blood in the needle and syringe, thus placing subsequent users of the injection equipment at risk.

In addition to booting, there is also *jacking*, a practice more common to cocaine injectors than to users of other injection drugs. Jacking is staged shooting:

> . . . that is, some injectors prefer to shoot the drug in stages rather than the full amount all at once. For example, if an IDU [injection drug user] has 50cc of dissolved cocaine, he or she might shoot 15cc and then pull 15cc of blood back into the syringe, wait for the rush to subside, inject 25cc and pull back 25cc of blood, wait again for the rush to pass, and then inject the remaining mix, perhaps jacking one more time to make sure no cocaine is left in the syringe.[26]

The booting/jacking process further increases the likelihood that traces of potentially infected blood remain in the needle/syringe, thus placing the next user at risk. Moreover, because of the way that injection equipment is cleaned and distributed in galleries, the potential for coming in contact with an infected needle/syringe is high. When the user has paid his or her fee to use the gallery, a needle/syringe is taken from those available on a table or in a container. In some galleries, the user is given a syringe by the gallery operator and has no choice in the matter. In either case, the equipment is not usually scrutinized for traces of blood, but rather for dull or clogged needles. Should such an impairment be evident, only then will the user return it for a substitute. Moreover, needles are generally not cleaned prior to use. "Shooting up" as quickly as possible is the matter of prime importance. After injecting and before returning the needle/syringe to the common container, the user is expected to rinse it—not necessarily for the sake of decontamination, but to prevent any drug/blood residue from hardening and causing an obstruction. Sometimes this rinsing is indeed done, but with water, which does not deactivate HIV. Sometimes the rinsing is done with infected water taken from a container to rinse other needles.

While systematic research and clinical observation suggest that the use of shooting galleries, the sharing of needles and other drug paraphernalia, and the practices of booting and jacking combine to explain the increasing proportion of injection drug users infected with HIV, little is known about the prevalence of HIV antibodies in needle/syringe combinations utilized by drug injectors. To study this subject, investigators took samples of needle/syringe combinations from major shooting galleries in Dade County (Miami), Florida. The samples were collected for the sake of analyzing their contents for the presence of HIV antibodies.[27]

Based on the investigators' knowledge of the Miami-Dade drug scene and the mapping of shooting gallery locations, three particular galleries were selected for study. All three were popular places in different geographical sectors of Miami. Site 1 was a three-bedroom house that had operated as a gallery since 1982 and as a *base house* (crack house) for the sale and smoking of crack-cocaine since 1985. Site 2 was a one-bedroom apartment in a two-family structure that had operated as a shooting gallery continuously since 1973. Site 3 was a single-room apartment in a 14-unit complex that had been established only recently as both a shooting gallery and base house. The three sites were located along a 15-mile arc, stretching from the vicinity of downtown Miami to the city's northwestern edge. Furthermore, the houses were located in areas having the county's highest rates of both drug use and crime.[28] According to U.S. Bureau of Census data, these areas were also characterized by high rates of unemployment, poor housing, infant mortality, teenage pregnancy, and low educational attainment.

Access to the three galleries was gained through the efforts of a staff field worker who had a variety of contacts in the Miami-Dade underground drug scene. Every morning during several one-week periods, each gallery was visited by the field worker who collected all the needles that had been used during the prior 24-hour period. Each site was paid a flat fee per visit regardless of the number of needles obtained. All needle/syringe combinations were labeled and visually graded as to condition: "clean" (if they contained no visible dirt, stains, or blood), "dirty" (if they contained dirt or stains but no visible blood), and "visible blood" (if they appeared to contain any liquid or dried blood). Of a total of 212 needle/syringe combinations collected, 62 could not be analyzed for the presence of HIV antibodies because of clogging, broken plungers, or other physical damage, leaving 150 available for laboratory analysis.*

Of the 150 needles tested, 15 were found to be seropositive (positive for HIV antibodies); 133 were seronegative; and in two cases serostatus was indeterminate. The overall seropositivity rate was 10 percent, with no significant differences between sites. In addition, although the number of customers frequenting these galleries tended to vary from one day to the next, further analysis demonstrated that there were no apparent distinctions in seropositivity rates by day of the week. However, a strong relationship was found between the graded condition of needle/syringe combinations and the presence of HIV antibodies. Of the 55 combinations graded as "clean" through visual inspection, only 5.5 percent were found to be seropositive, with a similar rate (4.7 percent) for "dirty" needles and syringes. By contrast, 20 percent of the needle/syringe combinations containing visible blood were found to be HIV positive. These data indicated a clearly significant relationship between the appearance of a needle/syringe and the presence of HIV antibodies. A "clean" needle/syringe had a significantly lesser chance of containing HIV antibodies. Conversely, one out of five needle/syringe combinations containing "visible blood" also contained HIV antibodies. Moreover, the data were indicative of the high rate of seropositivity among users of the three shooting galleries selected for this study and the high risk a user has in choosing a needle/syringe containing blood. Thus, it would appear that shooting galleries represent a significant health problem as far as the spread of the HIV infection is concerned. The operators of the galleries studied here reported that each serviced an average of 125 injection drug users per week, with many of the clients visiting more than once.

In a further attempt to understand the potential health risk of using needles and syringes in shooting galleries, consider the following,

---

*A pilot study was conducted with 17 sample needle/syringe combinations—10 samples containing HIV antibodies and seven nonreactive samples—to determine if HIV antibodies could actually be found in residue from needle/syringe combinations. The laboratory technician conducting the tests was unaware as to which needle/syringe combinations contained HIV antibodies, and the analysis accurately identified the 10 syringes through which blood containing HIV antibodies had been drawn. For a complete description of this effort, see Dale D. Chitwood, Clyde B. McCoy, James A. Inciardi, Duane C. McBride, Mary Comerford, Edward Trapido, H. Virginia McCoy, J. Bryan Page, James Griffin, Mary Ann Fletcher, and Margarita A. Ashman, "HIV Seropositivity of Needles from Shooting Galleries in South Florida," *American Journal of Public Health*, 80 (1990), pp. 1-3.

which suggests the probability of encountering a seropositive needle/syringe, given a 10 percent seropositivity rate and the shooting up totals of one to five times a day:

Number of Days Before There Is a 90 Percent Probability of a Seropositive Needle/Syringe Encounter at Varying Frequencies of Injection*

1x per day	22 days
2x per day	11 days
3x per day	7 days
4x per day	5 days
5x per day	4 days

* These probabilities must be examined with some caution, for they were computed on the basis of two assumptions: 1) an equal distribution of a 10 percent positivity rate across sites and days of the week; and, 2) a user's random selection of needles and syringes at the shooting gallery.

What all of this means is that given a 10 percent seropositivity rate, a user shooting up just once a day in a gallery would have a 90 percent chance of encountering an HIV-infected needle/syringe within 21.5 days. Shooting up three times a day in a gallery reduces the number of days to 7.17, and shooting up five times a day further reduces the time for a seropositive encounter to within 4.3 days.

The 10 percent seropositivity rate and the high probability of encountering an HIV-infected needle/syringe in a shooting gallery may help us to understand the high rates of HIV infection among injection drug users being reported in the literature. Further studies have demonstrated that the virus is actually culturable from needle/syringe combinations (which means that drug paraphernalia are indeed capable of transmitting living viral material),[29] and that water is an inappropriate medium for cleaning needles. Recent research at the University of Miami School of Medicine has documented that HIV is deactivated after a 30-second exposure to undiluted household bleach.[30]

CRACK-COCAINE, CRACK HOUSES, AND CRACK-HOUSE SEX

Although the potential for viral transmission is considerable in shooting galleries as the result of the multiple use of injection equipment, exchanges of sex for drugs are not particularly common. It happens, but not with great frequency. A female informant in Miami commented in 1992:

When I got to the place I was really sick [in withdrawal] and I didn't have enough dope to give away to anybody and still fix, but I know the house man would want a taste to let me fix there. So I told him, "Look, I don't have nothin' to give you, so how 'bout if I taste that." You know, I would give him head, a blow job. But he says, "Sure junkie, on your back!" He wanted to do a vaginal. So he let me in and we had sex, but he said it was okay only this time because there was nobody there. He doesn't like that sort of thing in his place when there are customers. He says that sexing in a get-off house has no class.*

This avoidance of sexual exchanges in shooting galleries is not unique to Miami. In Chicago, "cash galleries" are operated as businesses and charge from one to three dollars for admission; there are also "taste galleries," places where friends allow friends to use drugs, in exchange for a "taste," but where bartered sexual contacts are uncommon.[31] Operators of both types of galleries view the selling of sex as more trouble than it is worth. By contrast, however, sex-for-drugs exchanges are commonplace in many crack houses—in Miami, New York, Los Angeles, Denver, and elsewhere.

Crack-Cocaine

Crack is a variety of cocaine base, produced by "cooking" cocaine hydrochloride in water and baking soda. It has been called the "fast-food" variety of cocaine and is popular in the United States because it is cheap, easy to conceal, vaporizes with practically no odor, and provides swift gratification—a short-lived (up to five minutes) but nevertheless intense, almost sexual euphoria. Smoking cocaine as opposed to snorting it results in more immediate and direct absorption of the drug, producing a quicker and more compelling "high," greatly increasing the dependence potential. Moreover, there is increased risk of acute toxic reactions, including brain seizure, cardiac irregularities, respiratory paralysis, paranoid psychosis, and pulmonary dysfunction.[32]

Users typically smoke for as long as they have crack or the means to purchase it—money, personal belongings, sexual services, stolen goods, or other drugs. It is rare that smokers have but a single "hit" of crack. More likely they spend $50 to $500 during what they call a "mission"—a three or four day binge, during which they smoke almost constantly, three to 50 rocks per day. During these cycles, crack users rarely eat or sleep. And once crack is tried, for many users it is not long before it becomes a daily habit. The tendency to "binge" on crack for days at a time, neglecting food, sleep, and basic hygiene, severely compromises physical health. Consequently, crack users appear emaciated most of the time. They lose interest in their physical appearance.

---

*To complete the picture here, at the time of the contact with this woman in the street, she was an injection drug user, her husband was an injector, as was the "house man." Furthermore, she suspected that she was HIV positive, although she had never been tested. In addition, she was a street prostitute and used condoms with less than half of her clients.

Many have scabs on their faces, arms, and legs—the result of burns and picking at the skin (to remove bugs and other insects believed to be crawling *under* the skin). Crack users often have burned facial hair from carelessly lighting their smoking paraphernalia; they have burned lips and tongues from the hot stems of their pipes; and many seem to cough constantly.

Crack first became popular in many inner-city communities in the United States during the mid-1980s. Shortly after the drug was noticed by the media, press and television reports began describing crack use as an "epidemic" and "plague" that was devastating entire communities.[33] Considerable focus was placed on how the high-addiction liability of the drug instigated users to commit crimes to support their habits, on how youths were drawn into the crack-selling business, on how the violence associated with attempts to control crack distribution networks turned some communities into urban "dead zones" where crime was totally out of control, on how crack engendered a "hypersexuality" among users, and on how the drug was contributing to the further spread of HIV and AIDS.[34]

Researchers have documented that the alleged "hypersexuality" of crack users is most often played out within the confines of inner-city "crack houses." Crack houses are of numerous types.[35] Some are equipped with reinforced doors and walls, and their sole purposes are to manufacture and package crack. Others are all-purpose drug dens in which a variety of substances are available and in which some users inject heroin or cocaine while others smoke crack. A common type of crack or "base" house in many urban areas is a small apartment in which the primary activities are the making, selling, and smoking of crack. Sometimes there are exchanges of sex for crack.

Crack, Sexuality, and HIV Infection

Since the very beginnings of the crack "epidemic" in the United States, the drug has been viewed by many commentators as a sexual stimulant and enhancer, as well as the cause of "hypersexuality" in many users. Reports from the field and in the media have indicated that crack is the "ultimate turn-on"; that crack users readily engage in any variety of sexual activity, at any time and under any circumstances, and with an abundance of partners; that crack use has initiated a "new prostitution" and that the crack house has become the "new brothel"; and that the numerous rates of "sex-for-crack" exchanges in some locales were increasing the spread of HIV infection.[36]

To understand the crack phenomenon, one needs to realize the effects of the drug. First, cocaine's (and hence crack's) potent psychic dependence has been well documented.[37] Compulsive users seek the extreme mood elevation, elation, and grandiose feelings of heightened mental and physical prowess induced by the drug. When these begin to wane, a corresponding deep depression is felt, which is in such marked contrast to the users' previous states that they are strongly motivated to repeat the dose and restore their euphoria. Thus, when chronic users try to stop using crack, they are often plunged into a severe depression from which only the drug can arouse them.

Second, as an aphrodisiac, cocaine in either its powdered or base (crack) forms is problematic. Research has found considerable differences in sexual responses to the same dosage level of cocaine, depending primarily on the setting of the use and the background experiences of the user. Among recreational users, the male sexual response to cocaine is similar to that of women. For men, cocaine not only helps to prevent premature ejaculation, but at the same time permits prolonged intercourse before orgasm. Among women, achieving a climax under the influence of cocaine is often quite difficult. For both, however, when an orgasm finally occurs, it is quite explosive. Research findings also indicate that chronic, heavy users of cocaine, by contrast, typically experience sexual dysfunction.[38] Yet the association between crack use and apparent "hypersexual behaviors" has been evident in numerous ethnographic analyses of the crack scene.[39] Indeed, the tendency of crack users to engage in high-frequency sex with numerous, anonymous partners is a feature of crack dependence and crack-house life in many locales.

In support of these considerations, data were collected in Miami on the relationship between crack and sexuality, patterns of "sex-for-crack" exchanges, and their potential impact on the spread of HIV infection. Systematic interviews were conducted with 17 males and 35 females who were regular users of crack and who had exchanged sex for crack or for money to buy crack within the 30-day period prior to study recruitment. These interviews were conducted during the period November 1989 through June 1990, and the cases were drawn from the street by an experienced outreach worker and from a pool of recent admissions (within the previous 48 hours) to a local drug-treatment program. In addition, during the period September 1989 through February 1992, interviews and observations were conducted in several Miami crack houses. Additional insights were obtained from numerous contacts with other players in the local street subculture.*

Although the sample size and case selection procedures make generalization difficult, the data from both the structured and unstructured interviews clearly suggest that a great many persons who exchange sex for crack are not casual users of drugs. Most had been using illegal drugs for at least a decade, almost half had injected drugs

---

*For a fuller examination of this study, see James A. Inciardi, Dorthy Lockwood, and Anne E. Pottieger, *Women and Crack-Cocaine* (New York: Macmillan, 1993).

at some point in their drug-using careers, and virtually all were daily users of crack at the time of study recruitment. Similarly, exchanges of sex for money or drugs were not new experiences for these individuals. The interview and observational data suggest that individuals who exchange sex for crack do so with considerable frequency, and through a variety of sexual activities. The systematic data indicated that almost a third of the men and 89 percent of the women had had 100 or more sex partners during the 30-day period prior to study recruitment. Moreover, one of the key informants in the study reported having had more than 30,000 anonymous sexual contacts during the previous three years.

Many of the "clients" in the sex-for-crack exchanges were observed and interviewed in crack houses, and the overwhelming majority of these were chronic crack users who bartered crack with women and sometimes other men on a regular basis in return for sexual services. Much of this sexual activity occurred in crack houses, in a "freak" room—a bedroom in which the sexual activities occur. However, sex acts also occur in the more public smoking rooms as well.

The question is whether the crack–sex association is primarily pharmacological or sociocultural in nature. That is, do crack users exhibit hypersexual behavior because their drug provides hypersexual stimulation and enjoyment? Or is the aphrodisiac effect of crack a mythical explanation for behavior that actually results from economic and street-subculture factors? The best answer appears to be that both pharmacological and sociocultural factors are involved.

The pharmacological explanation of the crack–sex association begins with psychopharmacology: one effect of all forms of cocaine, including crack, is the release of normal inhibitions on behavior, including sexual behavior. The disinhibiting effect of cocaine is markedly stronger than that of depressants such as alcohol, Valium, or heroin. While the latter drugs typically cause a release from worry and an accompanying increase in self-confidence, cocaine typically causes elation and an accompanying gross overestimate of one's own capabilities. Further, since the effects of cocaine have a rapid onset, so too does the related release of inhibitions.

Medical authorities generally concede that because of the disinhibiting effects of cocaine, its use among new users does indeed enhance sexual enjoyment and improve sexual functioning, including the production of more intense orgasms.[40] These same reports maintain, however, that among long-term addicts, cocaine decreases both sexual desire and performance. Going further, the crack–sex association involves the need of female crack addicts to pay for their drug. Even this connection has a pharmacological component—crack's rapid onset, extremely short duration of effects, and high addiction liability combine to result in compulsive use and a willingness to obtain the drug through any means. In addition, although overdose is a constant threat, crack use does not pose the kind of physiological limit on the maximum needed (or possible) daily dosage. Whereas the heroin addict typically needs four doses a day, for example, and an alcoholic not uncommonly passes out after reaching a certain stage of intoxication, the heavy crack user typically uses until the supply is gone—be that minutes, hours, or days. The consequent financial burden can be staggering. Other parts of the economic crack–sex relationship, however, are strictly sociocultural. As in the legal job market, the access of women in the street subcultures to illegal income is typically more limited than is that of men. Prostitution has long been the easiest, most lucrative, and most reliable means for women to finance drug use.[41]

The combined pharmacological and sociocultural effects of crack use can put female users in severe jeopardy. Because crack makes its users ecstatic and yet is so short-acting, it has an extremely high addiction potential. Use rapidly becomes compulsive use. Crack acquisition thus becomes enormously more important than family, work, social responsibility, health, values, modesty, morality, or self-respect. This makes sex-for-crack exchanges psychologically tolerable as an economic necessity. Further, the disinhibiting effects of crack enable users to engage in sexual acts they might not otherwise even consider. For the female crack addict, the consequences may be extreme sexual behavior, but the term hypersexuality is very deceptive.

Going further, the lifestyle of crack users appears to increase their potential for exposure to HIV. Recent increases in the prevalence of other sexually transmitted diseases (STDs), particularly syphilis, have coincided with the advent of the crack epidemic,[42] and higher rates of sexually transmitted diseases have been identified among crack users than among non-users.[43] In addition, the prevalence of HIV in a number of locales has been found to be higher among crack users than among non-users.[44] The reasons for these higher rates of HIV infection are associated with the high frequency of sexual activity among crack users, their numerous sex partners, and their high potential for engaging in sex with intravenous drug users.*

POSTSCRIPT

For those who frequent bathhouses and sex clubs, or shooting galleries and crack houses, the risks for HIV infection are considerable. These locales, furthermore, have a few things in common.

---

*The potential for the heterosexual transmission of HIV through the bartering of sex for crack in crack houses is examined at length in Chapter Four.

In the gay baths and sex clubs, there is high-risk sex with numerous, anonymous sex partners. Virtually all visitors to the bathhouses are gay and bisexual men and are at high risk for HIV and AIDS through unprotected sex. And because the majority of those who engage in risky sex in the baths are frequent callers at these establishments, the potential for encountering an HIV-positive sex partner is considerable.

In the shooting galleries, there is needle sharing and the multiple use of injection paraphernalia, much of which is likely to be contaminated. Virtually all visitors to the galleries and get-offs are injection drug users, and they represent a major risk group for HIV and AIDS. Because the majority of those who share drug paraphernalia in shooting galleries do so on a regular basis, the potential for sharing with an infected partner is considerable.

In the crack houses, there is high-risk sex with numerous, anonymous sex partners, at least to the extent that these activities occur in bathhouses. Many of the women and men who exchange sex for crack are injection drug users, and many are prostitutes. Because the majority of those who exchange sex for crack in crack houses do so on a relatively frequent basis, the potential for encountering an HIV-infected partner is considerable.

Finally, with the exception of those men who have sex exclusively with other men, the majority of the visitors to the baths and sex clubs and to the shooting galleries and crack houses represent vectors for the spread of AIDS through heterosexual transmission.

END NOTES

1. Lloyd Morris, *Incredible New York* (New York: Bonanza Books, 1951), p. 324.

2. Paul Morand, *New York* (New York: William Heinemann, Ltd, 1930), p. 174.

3. See Walter Reckless, *Vice in Chicago* (Chicago: University of Chicago Press, 1933), pp. 120–136.

4. See Edward Winslow Martin, *Sins of the Great City: A Work Descriptive of the Virtues and Vices, the Mysteries, Miseries and Crimes of New York City* (Philadelphia: National, 1868); Herbert Asbury, *The Gangs of New York* (Garden City, NY: Garden City Publishing Co., 1928); Luc Sante, *Low Life: Lures and Snares of Old New York* (New York: Farrar, Straus, and Giroux, 1991).

5. For a lurid description of a hashish club, see H. H. Kane, "A Hashish–House in New York," *Harper's Monthly*, 67 (November 1883), pp. 944–949.

6. Fernando Henriques, *Prostitution in Europe and the Americas* (New York: Citadel Press, 1965); William W. Sanger, *The History of Prostitution: Its Extent, Causes and Effects Throughout the World* (New York: Medical Publishing Co., 1899).

7. "Playboy Interview: Larry Kramer," *Playboy*, September 1993, pp. 61–76.

8. *Playboy*, p. 64.

9. Larry Kramer, *Faggots* (New York: Random House, 1978).

10. Quoted in Leigh W. Rutledge, *The Gay Decades* (Plume Books, 1992), p. 129.

11. Larry Kramer, *Reports from the Holocaust: The Making of an AIDS Activist* (New York: St. Martin's Press, 1989), p. 6.

12. James Miller, "Dante on Fire Island: Reinventing Heaven in the AIDS Elegy," in Timothy F. Murphy and Suzanne Poirier (eds.), *Writing AIDS: Gay Literature, Language, and Analysis* (New York: Columbia University Press, 1993), pp. 265–305.

13. *Faggots*, p. 17.

14. *New York Native*, 16-29 July 1984, p. 23.

15. For detailed descriptions of the early gay bath scene, see Jim Marko, "After the Everard: A Look at Boston's Baths," *Gay Community News*, 18 June 1977, pp. 7–8; Edward W. Delph, *The Silent Community: Public Homosexual Encounters* (Beverly Hills: Sage Publications, 1978), pp. 135–148; Frances Fitzgerald, "The Castro-II," *The New Yorker*, 62 (28 July 1986), pp. 45–64; Martin S. Weinberg and Colin J. Williams, "Gay Baths and the Social Organization of Impersonal Sex," in Martin P. Levine (ed.), *Gay Men: The Sociology of Male Homosexuality* (New York: Harper & Row, 1979), pp. 164–181; Philip Weiss, "Inside a Bathhouse," *The New Republic*, 193 (2 Dec. 1985), pp. 12–13.

16. For a detailed examination of the bathhouse debate, see Ronald Bayer, *Private Acts, Social Consequences: AIDS and the Politics of Public Health* (New York: Free Press, 1989), pp. 20–71; Dennis Altman, *AIDS in the Mind of America: The Social, Political, and Psychological Impact of the New Epidemic* (New York: Doubleday, 1987); Randy Shilts, *And the Band Played*

On: Politics, People, and the AIDS Epidemic (New York: St. Martin's Press, 1987); *New York v. St. Mark's Baths*, New York Misc. Reports (2d Ser.) 130:911 (1986); Larry Gostin and William J. Curran, "Legal Control Measures for AIDS: Reporting Requirements, Surveillance, Quarantine, and Regulation of Public Meeting Places," *American Journal of Public Health*, 77 (1987), pp. 214–218; *Time*, 4 Nov. 1985, p. 25; *Maclean's*, 19 Nov. 1985, p. 52.

17. *The New York Times*, 5 March 1993, pp. B1, B5; *The New York Times*, 29 April 1993, p. B3; *Newsweek*, 11 Jan. 1993, pp. 60–61; *Miami Herald*, 12 Feb. 1991, p. 1C; *Miami Herald*, 24 June 1992, p. 3B; *Philadelphia Inquirer*, 31 May 1993, p. A1.

18. *The New York Times*, March 5, 1995, p. B5.

19. Charles Silverstein and Felice Picano, *The New Joy of Gay Sex* (New York: Harper/Collins, 1992), pp. 106–107.

20. Michael Agar, *Ripping and Running: A Formal Ethnography of Urban Heroin Addicts* (New York: Seminar Press, 1973); Seymour Fiddle, *Portraits From a Shooting Gallery* (New York: Harper & Row, 1967); Leroy Gould, Andrew L. Walker, Lansing E. Crane, and Charles W. Lidz, *Connections: Notes From the Heroin World* (New Haven: Yale University Press, 1974); Bill Hanson, George Beschner, James M. Walters, and Elliott Bovelle, *Life With Heroin: Voices From the Inner City* (Lexington, MA: D.C. Heath, 1985); Bruce D. Johnson, Paul J. Goldstein, Edward Preble, James Schmeidler, Douglas S. Lipton, Barry Spunt, and Thomas Miller, *Taking Care of Business: The Economics of Crime by Heroin Users* (Lexington, MA: D.C. Heath, 1985); Richard P. Rettig, Manual J. Torres, and Gerald R. Garrett, *Manny: A Criminal Addict's Story* (Boston: Houghton Mifflin, 1977); Sheigla Murphy and Dan Waldorf, "Kickin' Down to the Street Doc: Shooting Galleries in the San Francisco Bay Area," *Contemporary Drug Problems*, 18 (1991), pp. 9–29; J. Bryan Page, "Shooting Scenarios and Risk of HIV–1 Infection," *American Behavioral Scientist*, 33 (1990), pp. 478–490; J. Bryan Page, Dale D. Chitwood, Prince C. Smith, Normie Kane, and Duane C. McBride, "Intravenous Drug Abuse and HIV Infection in Miami," *Medical Anthropology Quarterly*, 4 (1989), pp. 57–72; J. Bryan Page, Prince C. Smith, and Normie Kane, "Shooting Galleries, Their Proprietors, and Implications for Prevention of AIDS," *Drugs and Society* 3 (1990), pp. 69–85.

21. Murphy and Waldorf, p. 12.

22. Hanson et al., p. 43.

23. James A. Inciardi, *Careers in Crime* (Chicago: Rand McNally, 1975), p. 53.

24. Murphy and Waldorf, p. 15.

25. Lawrence Greenfield, George E. Bigelow, and Robert K. Brooner, "HIV Risk Behavior in Drug Users: Increased Blood Booting During Cocaine Injection," *AIDS Education and Prevention*, 4 (1992), pp. 95–107.

26. Lawrence J. Ouellet, Antonio D. Jimenez, Wendell A. Johnson, and W. Wayne Wiebel, "Shooting Galleries and HIV Disease: Variations in Places for Injecting Illicit Drugs," *Crime and Delinquency*, 37 (1991), pp. 64–85.

27. Dale D. Chitwood, Clyde B. McCoy, James A. Inciardi, Duane C. McBride, Mary Comerford, Edward Trapido, H. Virginia McCoy, J. Bryan Page, James Griffin, Mary Ann Fletcher, and Margarita A. Ashman, "HIV Seropositivity of Needles from Shooting Galleries in South Florida," *American Journal of Public Health*, 80 (1990), pp. 1-3.

28. See Duane C. McBride and Clyde B. McCoy, "Crime and Drug Using Behavior: An Areal Analysis," *Criminology*, 19 (1981), pp. 281–302.

29. Edward J. Trapido, Clyde B. McCoy, Dale D. Chitwood, and L. Resnick, "HIV-1 Cultures From Shooting Gallery Needles and Syringes," *VI International Conference on AIDS*, San Francisco, 20-24 June 1990.

30. Paul Shapshak, Clyde B. McCoy, James E. Rivers, Dale D. Chitwood, Deborah C. Mash, Norman L. Weatherby, James A. Inciardi, Syed M. Shah, and Barry S. Brown, "Inactivation of Human Immunodeficiency Virus-1 at Short Time Intervals Using Undiluted Bleach," *Journal of Acquired Immune Deficiency Syndromes*, 6 (1993), pp. 218–219; Paul Shapshak, Clyde B. McCoy, Syed M. Shah, J. Bryan Page, James E. Rivers, Norman L. Weatherby, Dale D. Chitwood, and Deborah C. Mash, "Preliminary Laboratory Studies of Inactivation of HIV-1 in Needles and Syringes Containing Infected Blood Using Undiluted Household Bleach," *Journal of Acquired Immune Deficiency Syndromes*, 7 (1994), pp. 754–759.

31. Ouellet et al.

32. Barbara C. Wallace, *Crack Cocaine: A Practical Treatment Approach for the Chemically Dependent* (New York: Brunner/Mazel, 1991); James A. Inciardi, "Beyond Cocaine: Basuco, Crack, and Other Coca Products," *Contemporary Drug Problems*, 14 (1987), pp. 461–492; James A. Inciardi, *The War on Drugs II: The Continuing Epic of Heroin, Cocaine, Crack, Crime, AIDS, and Public Policy* (Mountain View, CA: Mayfield, 1992).

33. Inciardi, 1987.

34. See *The New York Times*, 29 Nov. 1985, pp. 1A, B6; *Newsweek*, 16 June 1986, pp. 15–22; *USA Today*, 16 June 1986, p. 1A; *Newsweek*, 30 June 1986, pp. 52–53; *The New York Times*, 25 Aug. 1986, pp. B1–B2; *The New York Times*, 24 Nov. 1986, pp. 1A, B2; *Newsweek*, 27 April 1987, pp. 35–36; *The New York Times*, 20 March 1988, p. E9; *Miami Herald* ("Neighbors" supplement), 24 April 1988, pp. 21–25; *The New York Times*, 23 June 1988, pp. A1, B4; *Time*, 5 Dec. 1988, p. 32; *New York Doctor*, 10 April 1989, pp. 1, 22; *U.S. News & World Report*, 10 April 1989, pp. 20–32.

35. Inciardi, *War on Drugs II*, pp. 117–124; Terry Williams, *Crackhouse: Notes From the End of the Line* (Reading, MA: Addison-Wesley, 1992; Phillipe Bourgois, "In Search of Horatio Alger: Culture and Ideology in the Crack Economy," *Contemporary Drug Problems*, 16 (1989), pp. 619–649; Ansley Hamid, "The Political Economy of Crack-Related Violence," *Contemporary Drug Problems*, 17 (1990), pp. 31–78; James A. Inciardi, "Kingrats, Chicken Heads, Slow Necks, Freaks, and Blood Suckers: A Glimpse at the Miami Sex for Crack Market," in Ratner, *Crack Pipe as Pimp*; Joseph B. Treaster, "Inside a Crack House: How Drug Use Is Changing," *The New York Times*, 6 April 1991, pp. 1, 10.

36. Mary Ann Chiasson, Rand L. Stoneburner, Deborah S. Hildebrandt, William E. Ewing, Edward E. Telsak, and Harold W. Jaffe, "Heterosexual Transmission of HIV-1 Associated With the Use of Smokable Freebase Cocaine (Crack)," *AIDS*, 5 (1991), pp. 1121–1126; Mindy Thompson Fullilove and Robert E. Fullilove, "Intersecting Epidemics: Black Teen Crack Use and Sexually Transmitted Disease," *Journal of the American Women's Medical Association*, 44 (1989), pp. 146–153; Charisse L. Grant, "Life Goes on Along Crack Bazaar," *Miami Herald*, 31 May 1988, pp. 1B, 2B; Frank Greve, "Sex Effect of Cocaine Its Biggest Turn–on?" *Miami Herald*, 22 Oct. 1989, pp. 1G, 6G; Philip J. Hilts, "Spread of AIDS by Heterosexuals," *The*

New York Times, 1 May 1990, pp. C1, C12; James A. Inciardi, "Trading Sex for Crack Among Juvenile Drug Users: A Research Note," *Contemporary Drug Problems,* 16 (1989), pp. 689–700.

37. Arnold M. Washton and Mark S. Gold, *Cocaine: A Clinician's Handbook* (New York: Guilford Press, 1987).

38. Patrick T. Macdonald, Dan Waldorf, Craig Reinarman, and Sheigla Murphy, "Heavy Cocaine Use and Sexual Behavior," *Journal of Drug Issues,* 18 (1988), pp. 437–455.

39. See Mitchell S. Ratner (ed.), *Crack Pipe as Pimp: An Ethnographic Investigation of Sex-for-Crack Exchanges* (New York: Lexington Books, 1993).

40. Lester Grinspoon and James B. Bakalar, *Cocaine: A Drug and Its Social Evolution* (New York: Basic Books, 1985); Roger D. Weiss and Steven M. Mirin, *Cocaine* (Washington, DC: American Psychiatric Press, 1987).

41. Paul J. Goldstein, *Prostitution and Drugs* (Lexington, MA: D. C. Heath, 1979).

42. M. E. Guinan, "Women and Crack Addiction," *Journal of the American Women's Medical Association,* 44 (1989), p. 129; S. Schultz, M. Zweig, T. Sing, and M. Htoo, "Congenital Syphilis: New York City, 1986–1988," *American Journal of the Diseases of Children,* 144 (1990), p. 279.

43. R. T. Rolfs, M. Goldberg, and R. G. Sharrar, "Risk Factors for Syphilis: Cocaine Use and Prostitution," *American Journal of Public Health,* 80 (1990), pp. 853–857; Robert E. Fullilove, Mindy T. Fullilove, Benjamin P. Bowser, and S. A. Gross, "Risk of Sexually Transmitted Disease Among Black Adolescent Crack Users in Oakland and San Francisco, California," *Journal of the American Medical Association,* 263 (1990), pp. 851–855.

44. Benjamin P. Bowser, "Crack and AIDS: An Ethnographic Impression," *Journal of the National Medical Association,* 81 (1989), pp. 538–540; Claire Sterk, "Cocaine and HIV Seropositivity," *Lancet,* 7 May 1988, pp. 1052–1053; Edward J. Trapido, Nancy Lewis, and Mary Comerford, "HIV-1 and AIDS in Belle Glade, Florida: A Reexamination of the Issues," *American Behavioral Scientist* 33 (1990), pp. 451–464.

CHAPTER FOUR

The Heterosexual Transmission of HIV

B ack on July 26, 1983, the number of confirmed AIDS cases known to the Centers for Disease Control was comparatively few—some 1,922. Although the scientific community at that time was no longer referring to the new disease as G.R.I.D. or the "gay plague," the mechanisms of transmission were still not fully understood. The majority of these 1,922 cases, 71 percent, fell into what were referred to then as "risk groups"—gay and bisexual men, followed by intravenous drug users, Haitians, and hemophiliacs. As illustrated in Figure I, however, these "risk groups" were not mutually exclusive: there were gay and bisexual men who were intravenous drug users, there were gay and bisexual Haitians and hemophiliacs, and there were Haitians and hemophiliacs who were also drug injectors.

These overlapping cases were members of what have been called "bridging" groups—those whose multiple risk factors increased their likelihood of acquiring HIV in the first place as well as of transmitting it from one population group to another. Perhaps most notable in this bridging phenomenon were the 113 AIDS cases in Figure I designated as "all others"—those outside of the typical "high risk groups." The overwhelming majority of these individuals were the heterosexual partners of infected bisexual men, intravenous drug users, and hemophiliacs. The remainder included the infant children of HIV-infected mothers. Also, as AIDS became better understood it became clear that being "Haitian" did not place someone at a higher risk for AIDS infection. Rather, the concentration within that national group was the result of heterosexual transmission. Currently, of the 360,000 cumulative adult/adolescent AIDS cases reported to the Centers for Disease Control and Prevention through the close of 1993, 7 percent were the result of heterosexual contact.[1]

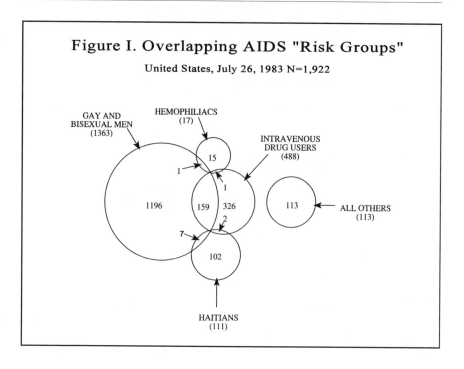

Figure I. Overlapping AIDS "Risk Groups"

United States, July 26, 1983 N=1,922

THE MECHANISMS OF HETEROSEXUAL TRANSMISSION

At present, the biological variables that determine HIV "infectivity" (the tendency to spread from host to host) and "susceptibility" (the tendency for a host to become infected) are incompletely understood. HIV has been isolated from the semen of infected men, and it appears that it may be harbored in the cells of pre-ejaculated fluids or sequestered in inflammatory lesions.[2] Furthermore, there is evidence that women can harbor HIV in vaginal and cervical secretions at varying times during the menstrual cycle.[3]

The probability of sexual transmission of HIV among gay and bisexual men through anal intercourse and to women through vaginal intercourse has been well documented.[4] However, although there is the potential for viral transmission from female secretions, the absolute amounts of virus in these secretions appear to be relatively low. The efficiency of transmission of male-to-female versus female-to-male is likely affected by the relative infectivity of these different secretions, as well as by the occurrence of sex during menses, specific sexual practices, the relative integrity of skin and mucosal surfaces involved, and the presence of other sexually transmitted diseases. Given these factors, there are a number of issues to be examined when considering the heterosexual transmission of HIV from men to women and from women to men. Of particular interest are the biological variables, risk factors and cofactors, and particular sexual practices among those populations with the highest rates of heterosexual transmission.

Before proceeding, however, it might be useful to examine the possible pathways along the heterosexual AIDS bridge. As illustrated in Figure II, the transmission points are several:

1. from gay and bisexual injection drug users to male and female heterosexual injection drug users through the sharing of drugs and/or injection equipment;

2. from male injection drug users to female injection drug users through sexual contact and the sharing of drugs and/or injection equipment;

3. from male injection drug users to female non-injectors through sexual contact;

4. from female injection drug users to male injection drug users through sexual contact and the sharing of drugs and/or injection equipment;

5. from female injection drug users to male non-injectors through sexual contact; and,

6. from males and females infected by their sex partners to other, subsequent sex partners.

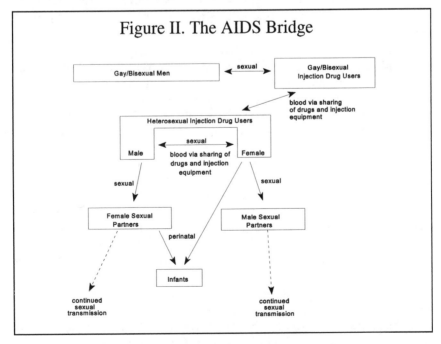

Figure II. The AIDS Bridge

Male-to-Female Transmission of HIV

Heterosexual contact per se is an *essential* but not necessarily *sufficient* condition for the transmission of HIV. A variety of studies have demonstrated, for example, that an average of only 15 percent of the women who are steady partners of HIV-infected men acquire the infection, despite repeated sexual exposures.[5] Thus, the risk of contracting HIV through a single sexual exposure is not particularly high in the great majority of instances.[6] However, there is evidence that although some people remain uninfected after hundreds of episodes of unprotected sex, others have become infected after only one or just a few sexual encounters.[7] These observations would suggest that there are cofactors that affect the likelihood of HIV transmission.

Three groups of factors influencing the probability of acquiring HIV through male-to-female sexual contact have been suggested: 1) sexual behavior and risk duration; 2) infectiousness of the HIV-positive partner; and, 3) host susceptibility.[8] Looking first at sexual behavior and risk duration, it has been noted in Chapter Two that the potential for infection among homosexuals increases with the number of partners and the frequency of sexual intercourse. However, a majority of early studies of heterosexual transmission failed to show a relationship between risk of infection and either the frequency of sexual intercourse or the duration of a relationship with an infected partner.[9] These results were surprising and counterintuitive and may have been the result of measurement error, improper statistical analysis, and the failure to account for other factors.

More recent investigations have found that the number of exposures to an infected partner is indeed associated with transmission. Important findings in this regard came from the California Partners' Study, an investigation that surveyed the opposite sex partners of individuals infected with HIV or diagnosed with AIDS.[10] Of 150 female partners of infected men recruited during the second half of the 1980s, 48 percent were partners of bisexual men, 15 percent were partners of injection drug users, 23 percent were partners of hemophiliacs, 5 percent were partners of men infected through contaminated blood transfusions, 5 percent were partners of men in multiple risk groups, and 4 percent were partners of men in unidentified risk groups. Of the 85 women who had had 0 to 200 sexual contacts with their infected partners, 13 percent were HIV positive; of the 65 women who had had 201 to 2,170 sexual contacts with their infected partners, 37 percent were HIV positive.

With regard to the infectiousness of the seropositive partner, a higher rate of infection among the female partners of men in advanced clinical stages of HIV disease has been well documented.[11] This is likely due to the fact that the declining immune function allows the virus to replicate, unchecked, in an HIV-positive individual, and as such, there are higher concentrations of HIV (termed "virus load") in such bodily fluids as blood and semen.

One of the more comprehensive studies of male-to-female sexual transmission examining the full range of risk behaviors was conducted by the Italian Study Group on HIV Heterosexual Transmission.[12] The sample included 368 women, 27.7 percent of whom were seropositive, whose only potential exposure to HIV was having a male sex partner who was HIV positive. The findings of the study documented risk duration, type and frequency of sexual intercourse, the man's infectiousness, and the woman's susceptibility as the key factors. In terms of risk duration, for example, women having a relationship with an infected male for one to five years had the highest prevalence of seropositivity, and a frequency of sexual intercourse more than twice a week was associated with a twofold increased risk of infection. Seropositive women reported anal intercourse twice as frequently as seronegative women, but condom use had a clear association with reduced rates of heterosexual transmission. In addition, infected women were more frequently those whose partners' disease had progressed to AIDS. Finally, seropositive women also reported histories of syphilis, genital warts, or genital herpes in greater proportion than seronegative women.

These studies document that although the transmission of HIV between male and female partners is not always certain with any given exposure, considerable risk is always present in either direction, and can increase dramatically depending on the type and frequency of the sexual contacts, and the immunological state of the partners.

The Efficiency of Female-to-Male Transmission

Female-to-male sexual transmission of HIV is supported by biological plausibility, equal numbers of male and female AIDS cases in some African countries, case reports of males with no risk factors other than heterosexual intercourse, and seroconversion of male sex partners of infected women that occurred while the couples were being studied prospectively. In terms of the biological plausibility of female-to-male transmission, it has been argued that since other sexually transmitted diseases are bidirectional in nature, it is not unreasonable to assume that HIV can spread in the same manner. A number of studies have documented that African and Indian men who have multiple female sex partners or sexual contact with prostitutes are at high risk for becoming infected with HIV.[13] The most persuasive case reports of female-to-male transmission have been those in which 1) the female acquired the infection from a transfusion or organ transplant and her male partner (without other known risk factors) subsequently seroconverted,[14] and 2) where a sequential chain of male-to-female-to-male transmission was observed.[15]

Although significant numbers of female-to-male infections have been documented in Africa,[16] such a mode of transmission has been reported only infrequently in the United States, and the majority of the more recent case reports have come from investigators in Europe.[17] Several explanations have been offered for the differences in female-to-male transmission rates between the United States and Africa. A number of researchers have suggested that the infrequent documentation of heterosexual transmission from women to men in this country may be a function of the history of the epidemic. They suggest that the initial phase was largely confined to male homosexuals and intravenous drug users, so that during that time the number of infected women was low, and the possibility of female-to-male transmission was small.

Because the majority of AIDS cases occurring today reflect infections that were acquired during the early years of the epidemic, most heterosexually acquired infections among men may still be in the asymptomatic or latent stage.[18] It has been added to this hypothesis, as noted earlier, that the infectivity of an HIV carrier increases over time, suggesting that this additional factor in the natural history of HIV infection may magnify the effects alluded to above. Following this line of reasoning, it has been argued that virus concentration in genital secretions may also increase over the course of the infection.[19] On the other hand, researchers from the National Institute on Drug Abuse have argued that the relative frequency of female-to-male transmission has been underestimated (primarily as the result of the way that cases are classified), suggesting that it represents a more significant public health concern than is generally believed.[20]

Of additional significance here are the relationships among prostitution, untreated sexually transmitted diseases (STDs), condom use, and HIV infection. In 1988, one group of researchers argued as follows:

> If prostitutes [in the United States] are effectively transmitting the AIDS virus to their customers, there would be far more cases of white, heterosexual males diagnosed with AIDS than are reflected in the current statistics, because some IVDUs in New York, including some prostitutes, have been infected with the AIDS virus since at least 1978. The average street prostitute sees 1,500 customers a year. If even five percent of female street prostitutes in New York City were infected by 1981, the year AIDS was first identified, even moderately efficient transmission of the virus from prostitutes to clients would have resulted in the diagnosis of at least 100,000 white, heterosexual men by now.[21]

In 1992, at an AIDS research planning meeting at the National Institute on Drug Abuse, the same argument was reiterated:

Direct information on customers becoming infected by sex workers is very limited, but does not support more than rare instances of transmission. CDC data report very low rates of "heterosexual transmission" or "no identified risk" of AIDS cases among men; given the number of men who purchase sex in this country, these low rates argue against anything but rare transmission.[22]

In Africa, by contrast, and as already noted, there is considerable evidence of viral transmission by HIV-infected prostitutes to their male customers.[23] A number of factors contribute to this difference. Among African prostitutes and their customers, there appear to be significant proportions with untreated STDs, including genital ulcers, and these appear to increase men's susceptibility to HIV.[24] In addition, several studies have noted that sex workers in the United States are more conscious of STDs and are more likely to use safer sexual practices (e.g., vaginal and anal sex with condoms) with customers than their counterparts in Africa.[25] For example, a number of reports have noted that there is a socialization process associated with becoming a prostitute in the United States. Would-be and neophyte prostitutes learn the appropriate sex industry techniques and safeguards through apprenticeships with pimps and/or more experienced prostitutes.[26]

In some cases, there is informal or even formal training on how to protect oneself from theft, violence, or disease. For example, in one sociological analysis of prostitution as an occupation, it was found that the recognition of sexually transmitted diseases was a specific topic of instruction for neophyte house prostitutes.[27] Furthermore, however loose, unstructured, and transitory their relationships may often be, those who work the streets or in organized houses of prostitution in the United States have friendships and peer relationships through which experiences are shared, techniques are traded, warnings are communicated, and knowledge is reinforced. Interestingly, however, what may be characteristic of "street walkers" and most other categories of prostitutes is not necessarily the case among those women and men who exchange sex for crack-cocaine.

HETEROSEXUAL TRANSMISSION AND THE BARTERING OF SEX FOR CRACK

The properties and effects of crack-cocaine, the cocaine/sexuality connection, and the characteristics of crack houses have already been described in Chapter Three. However, a number of these topics are revisited and expanded upon here since many of the considerations described in the preceding section have relevance to an understanding of sex-for-crack exchanges and their potential for the heterosexual transmission of HIV.

Crack and Sexually Transmitted Diseases

Although the bartering of sex for crack had been mentioned in the popular media at the very beginnings of the crack "epidemic,"[28] the first empirical study of the phenomenon did not appear in the scientific literature until 1989. In that analysis, drawn from a larger study of drug use and street crime among serious delinquents in Miami, the potential for HIV acquisition and transmission through sex-for-crack exchanges was addressed.[29] Of 100 girls in the 14-to-17-year age range, 27 had bartered sex-for-crack during the one-year period prior to interview. Of these, 11 had traded sex for drugs on fewer than six occasions, but had exchanged sex for money on an aggregate of 6,850 occasions. By contrast, there were others in the sample who had bartered sex hundreds and even thousands of times.

At about the same time that this study was being reported, several observers began to notice rising rates of syphilis and other sexually transmitted diseases among crack users.[30] Shortly thereafter, sex-for-crack exchanges were targeted for systematic study. However, one of the difficulties in assessing the nature of HIV risks associated with crack use is the fact that most crack users engage in multiple risk behaviors.

A study of risk factors for HIV infection was conducted at an STD clinic in an area in New York City where the cumulative incidence of AIDS in adults through mid-1990 was 9.1 per 1,000 population and where the use of illicit drugs, including crack smoking, was common.[31] The overall seroprevalence among the 3,084 volunteer subjects was 12 percent, with 80 percent of these seropositives reporting risk behaviors associated with HIV infection, including male-to-male sexual contact, intravenous drug use, and heterosexual contact with an injection drug user (IDU). The seroprevalence in individuals denying these risks was 3.6 percent in men (50 of 1,389) and 4.2 percent in women (22 of 522). Among these individuals, the behaviors associated with infection were prostitution and the use of crack in women and a history of syphilis, crack use, and sexual contact with a crack-using prostitute in men.

The potential for a male in sex-for-crack exchanges to come into contact with an HIV-positive female partner was demonstrated in a study of 87 New York City women who had been admitted to a municipal hospital with a diagnosis of pelvic inflammatory disease.[32] Crack use was reported by 56 percent of the subjects (N = 49), and of these, 20 percent were HIV seropositive. Crack use was significantly related to both "traditional" AIDS risk behaviors (injecting drugs and sex with an IDU) and other unsafe sexual behaviors (exchanging sex for money or drugs and having casual sex partners).

In 1989, given the potential of sex-for-crack exchanges for spreading HIV to new populations, the National Institute on Drug Abuse supported ethnographic studies of the phenomenon in eight cities—Chicago, Denver, Los Angeles, Miami, Newark, New York, Philadelphia, and San Francisco.[33] A total of 340 crack users were interviewed in depth (69 percent of whom were women). Of the 233 women, 108 had participated in sex-for-crack exchanges, as did 69 of the men. HIV testing was done with 168 of the subjects, and a total of 14 percent were found to be positive for HIV antibodies. Interestingly, of the 24 males who were non-injectors and who had engaged in heterosexual sex-for-crack exchanges, 12 percent were HIV positive.

The significance of crack use in the intensification of behavioral risks and the potential for HIV infection is dramatically illustrated in a recent report from researchers at the University of Miami School of Medicine.[34] Data for the analysis were drawn from the Miami Community Outreach Study, one of the many National AIDS Demonstration Research (NADR) projects funded by the National Institute on Drug Abuse during the closing years of the 1980s.

In this study, 1,359 injection drug users and their primary female sex partners were recruited from Miami's inner-city streets, assessed for their AIDS-related behavioral risks, tested for the presence of HIV antibodies, and placed into AIDS prevention/intervention programs. Within this sample, there were 235 women who had never injected drugs. These women were the focus of the analysis, and 40.9 percent of them had used crack while 59.1 percent had not.

There were significant differences in behavoral risks between these crack-using and non-using women. For example, the exchange of sex for money was reported by 64.5 percent of crack users and 18.4 percent of non-users. This difference was even more pronounced when exchanges of sex for drugs are considered—reported by 24.2 percent of the crack users but only 2.7 percent of non-users. Both groups of women had a high degree of HIV risk associated with having sex partners who were injection drug users—90 percent of the non-crack users and 96 percent of the crack users, but this was an expected finding since the study had targeted drug injectors and their sex partners from the outset. Both groups, furthermore, reported an infrequent use of condoms. Going further, crack users reported a mean of 13.6 sex partners in the past month, while non-crack users reported only 1.6. There was less difference in the number of injecting sex partners, with crack users reporting a mean of 2.1 and non-crack users reporting 1.2.

Most notably, seropositivity for HIV was 19.8 percent among crack-using women and 10.8 percent among the non-users. As such, it would appear that crack puts women at greater risk for contracting HIV infection, and that the source of the risk lies in the apparently strong relationship between crack use and sexual behavior. Some confirmation for this hypothesis can be found in crack users' higher rates of other sexually transmitted diseases. The STD found most common among study subjects was gonorrhea, reported by 42.7 percent of the crack users compared to 23.7 percent of the non-users. Similarly, syphilis was reported by 30.2 percent of the crack users, compared with 13.8 percent of the non-users, while genital sores were reported by 17.7 percent and 6 percent, respectively. Consequently, the relationships among crack use, unsafe sex, and injection drug use suggest that the use of crack-cocaine may increase heterosexual transmission of HIV among crack users, drug injectors, the sex partners of both groups, and outward from crack-using and drug-injecting networks to other populations.

Crack, Sex, and the Spread of HIV

As noted earlier in this chapter, the sexual transmission of HIV from men to women appears to be more pronounced than that of women to men. However, the potential for transmission of HIV from women to men with no other risk factors within the context of sex-for-crack exchanges is quite possible, and is related to a number of considerations, including two important independent risk factors. The first is the cocaine/sexuality connection, described at length in Chapter Three. Cocaine has long had a reputation as an aphrodisiac, although sexuality is notoriously a playground of legend, exaggeration, and rumor. In all likelihood, much of cocaine's reputation may be from the mental exhilaration and disinhibition it engenders, thus bringing about some heightened sexual pleasure during the early stages of use. At the same time, cocaine users have consistently reported that the drug tends to delay the sexual climax, and that after prolonged stimulation, an explosive orgasm occurs. Users also report that chronic use of the drug results in sexual dysfunction, with impotence and the inability to ejaculate being the common complaints of male users, the inability to climax among females, and decreased desire for sex becoming the norm for both male and female users.[35]

What applies to powder-cocaine with regard to sexual stimulation and functioning would also apply to crack-cocaine. Curiously, however, there is the rather contradictory evidence that crack appears to engender what has been referred to as "hypersexual" behavior among many users. This has been observed in a number of ethnographic studies.[36] Many crack-addicted women and men engage in any manner of sexual activity, under *any* circumstances, in private or in public, and with multiple partners of either sex (or both sexes simultaneously). Indeed, the tendency of some crack users to engage in high-frequency sex with numerous anonymous partners is a feature of crack dependence and crack-house life in many locales. Furthermore, sex-for-drugs exchanges seem to be far more common among female crack addicts now than they ever were among female narcotics addicts, even at the height of the 1967-1974 heroin epidemics.[37]

Crack-using male customers involved in sex-for-crack exchanges, although consistently reporting difficulties in maintaining an erection and ejaculating under the influence of the drug, state that sex, and particularly oral sex, while smoking not only enhances the drug's effects, but also gives them a sense of power and control that they typically do not have in other aspects of their lives.[38] For example, in 1990 a 40-year-old Miami male crack user/dealer reported:

> I've been shit on all my life, first by my parents and teachers and now by everybody. Fuck! Everybody seems to be always kickin' me in the ass. I can't even get laid without catchin' a lot o' shit. But fuck! The cracks puts me in charge of things. With the cracks I can get people to do things. For crack I can get women to do anything. And fuck, gettin' the brains [oral sex] while smokin' a rock is the best thing in the world. The best thing in the world. The best thing ever, anywhere.

Similarly, some women crack users also report an affinity for oral sex while smoking. A 36-year-old women who had been a crack user since the drug was first noticed in Miami in the early 1980s reported in 1992:

> I know it's weird and hard to explain, but it's true, crack and oral sex go together. Men like it and women like it, and maybe for the same reasons. I like it because if my partner does it slow and gentle, it's soothing, it sort of smooths off the rough edges. It just makes me feel good, and makes the drug better, and because I'm so high most of the time I don't much care if anyone is watching. It's a good thing.

A second independent risk factor relates to the impact of crack use on physical health and hygiene. As mentioned in Chapter Three, because of the pharmacology and addiction potential of crack, it is rare that smokers have but a single "hit" of the drug. Rather, they binge for days at a time, neglecting food, sleep, and basic hygiene. As a result, their physical health becomes severely compromised. In addition, mouth ulcerations and burned lips and tongues from the hot stems of the pipes are not uncommon, and many smokers have self-reported and have been observed to have untreated STDs.[39]

Going further, although street prostitutes who barter sex for money to purchase drugs often insist that their customers use condoms, this is not usually the case with crack house-sex. In fact, condoms are rarely seen in crack houses. Given the health status of crack users (including a high likelihood of compromised immune systems), the incidence of STDs (many of which go untreated), and general lack of condom use, many of the conditions that have contributed to the heterosexual transmission of HIV in Africa exist in crack houses in Miami, New York, Philadelphia, and other urban areas across the United States. In addition, given the frequency of sex and the large number of partners associated with crack-house sex, the potential for coming into contact with HIV is of an even greater magnitude. It is within this context that the heterosexual transmission of HIV is most likely.

Furthermore, a number of situations may make the crack house unique in the heterosexual spread of HIV. In a study of crack-house sexual activities in Miami, for example, a number of men reported that they could climax only through extremely vigorous masturbation or prolonged vaginal intercourse. Many of the female partners in these exchanges reported that the lengthy intercourse resulted in both vaginal and penile bleeding.[40] In situations such as these, the potential for female-to-male transmission of HIV increases. During vaginal intercourse, the friction of the penis against the clitoris, labia minora, and vaginal vestibule, opening, and canal causes stimulation that can generate copious amounts of vaginal secretions. And, as indicated previously in this chapter, HIV has been isolated from vaginal/cervical secretions. Moreover, since women who exchange sex-for-crack in crack houses do so with many different men during the course of a day or night, potentially HIV-infected semen from a previous customer can still be present in the vagina. It was reported by one crack house customer that he had ruptured the skin on his penis while having intercourse with a "crack-house prostitute" while she was menstruating. This informant also indicated that vaginal sex during menses was not a rare event. As such, genital secretions as well as semen and blood come into direct contact with the traumatized skin of a client's penis during crack-house sex.

In many crack houses, it is not uncommon for women to engage in repeated oral, vaginal, and anal sexual activities, often with no time lapse between successive customers. Since condom use is rare, not only are the women exposed to the semen of *all* of their male partners, but successive male partners also are exposed to the semen of the women's previous partners.[41] As such, *heterosexual transmission of HIV can be from male-to-female, female-to-male, and male-to-male.* It would appear, moreover, that this phenomenon is not unique to crack-house sex. In an Orange County, California, study of undocumented Hispanic migrant workers and heroin-addicted prostitutes,[42] a parallel situation was found. Large numbers of men engaged in vaginal intercourse with the same woman, in rapid succession—a sexual behavior referred to by the participants as becoming "milk brothers."

Finally, there is the matter of oral sex. Few studies have associated oro-genital sex with HIV transmission,[43] and the majority of reports have examined this transmission route among homosexual men.[44] Only one fully documented case of female-to-male transmission through oral sex has appeared in the literature.[45] In crack houses, oral sex (both fellatio and cunnilingus) is common. Given such risk factors and co-factors as STD infections, genital ulcers, lesions on the lips and tongue, and abrasions on the penis and in the vagina among those who exchange sex-for-crack, the potential for female-to-male transmission of HIV through oral sex is not inconsiderable.

PROSTITUTION AND HETEROSEXUAL TRANSMISSION

In 1984, when AIDS was still viewed as a disease generally limited to gay and bisexual men, intravenous drug users, hemophiliacs, and Haitians, the notion of heterosexual transmission was hardly considered. The opinion of the Centers for Disease Control on the matter at that time was terse and to the point:

> [T]he importance of female-to-male transmission of AIDS in the United States and the role, if any, of female prostitutes in this transmission have *not* been established.[46]

Serious discussion of the topic began the following year, however, when Dr. Harry W. Haverkos of the National Institute of Allergy and Infectious Diseases commented in a letter to the *Journal of the American Medical Association* that "female-to-male transmission [of AIDS] is highly likely," and that female prostitutes were contributing to the increasing rate of heterosexual transmission.[47] Other scientists quickly responded, suggesting that Haverkos was incorrect in his contention,[48] and the debate was on. By the close of 1985, the controversy had surfaced in the national press. In *The New York Times*, for example:

> A scientific debate has emerged over whether prostitutes are likely to spread AIDS among heterosexuals, a group that has largely been spared by the nation's AIDS epidemic up until now. Many scientists . . . say the fear that prostitutes will be a major conduit [of the disease] into the heterosexual community is unjustified.

> Other scientists believe that consorting with prostitutes has already caused some cases of AIDS in men, and that if current trends continue, prostitutes could transmit the virus to many men, who in turn will infect their unsuspecting wives and lovers.[49]

None of the principles in the debate expected the virus to course through the heterosexual population to the degree that it was devastating homosexual and intravenous drug-using communities. Nevertheless, there was evidence that heterosexual transmission was bidirectional in nature. In one study, both prostitutes and their clients in several African countries were found to be infected with HIV.[50] Given the conflicting opinions, are prostitutes indeed agents of the heterosexual spread of AIDS?

Prostitution and AIDS in the United States

In the United States, there appear to be a number of sides to the HIV/prostitution enigma. The first is that, in all likelihood, the proportion of American men having sexual contacts with prostitutes is statistically small. This is suggested by indicators of sexual activity in a household probability study conducted by the Institute for Survey Research at Temple University in 1990.[51] For example, 77.4 percent of the men in the survey reported having only one sex partner in the past year, and 81.4 percent reported having only one partner in the past 30 days. Furthermore, only 4.4 percent of the married men reported having a sex partner other than their spouse in the last year and only 1.8 percent reported this information for the past 30 days. Going further, a corroboration of these findings can be found in data from the 1991 Survey of Men conducted by the Battelle Memorial Institute with a nationally representative sample of men ages 20 to 39.[52] For example, 70.9 percent reported having only one sex partner since January 1990, and 95.8 percent of the married men reported only one partner in the same period.

In interpreting these data, a number of things must be kept in mind. Initially, since the samples were drawn from stable, at-home populations, they may have missed many members of higher-risk populations who have more numerous sex partners. On the other hand, in both studies there were many men who had had no sexual contacts—5.7 percent in the past year in the Temple survey and 4.3 percent since January 1990 in the Battelle survey. In addition, and perhaps most importantly, having more than one sex partner does not necessarily mean having sex with prostitutes. As such, it can be concluded from these data that the proportion of American men patronizing prostitutes is statistically small.

The second issue is whether prostitution in the United States is a significant risk factor for HIV and AIDS. The available evidence would suggest that it is not. A significant study in this regard included 78 predominantly white "call girls" and women working for escort services and massage parlors in New York City.[53] The women had been prostitutes for an average of five years, and each had had an average of over 200 clients during the past year, or approximately 1,000 lifetime partners. Among them, vaginal intercourse was common, anal sex was rare, and the use of condoms was at best sporadic. Six of these prostitutes had histories of intravenous drug use, but none of the remaining 72 had any other recognized risk factors for HIV infection. Interestingly, only one of the drug-injecting women was found to be HIV positive, and none of the 72 non-drug-abusers was positive for HIV.

Similar results were found in a series of studies of hundreds of street prostitutes in New York City conducted during the 1980s.[54] Overall, only 4.5 percent of the prostitutes were found to be HIV positive. However, there was an interesting and statistically significant finding: the HIV-positive women had a mean of 3,062 sex partners in their lifetimes, whereas the HIV-negatives had a mean of 1,047 lifetime partners. Furthermore, among those with histories of drug abuse, almost 50 percent were seropositive for HIV antibodies. This finding targets the third aspect of the prostitute/AIDS enigma, that drug abuse places someone at greater risk for HIV infection than prostitution. This finding suggests that overall susceptibility to infection may be more important in determining who becomes infected than is simple exposure to the virus.

Prostitution and AIDS in Other Countries

The facts surrounding the emergence of prostitution around the world are buried in antiquity, although its presence in human society was documented as early as biblical times.[55] There is evidence, furthermore, that prostitution has been a common enterprise in many cultures and societies down through the millennia.[56] Current observers suggest that poverty, social and economic chaos, and porous borders (with people easily moving back and forth) have recently turned commercial sex into a global growth industry:

> From Eastern Europe to the Himalayas, from Tokyo to Tegucigalpa, transaction by sordid transaction has created a multi-billion-dollar sex trade. It is encouraged by massive socioeconomic movements: the collapse of the Soviet empire, the increase in global mobility, the wrenching disparity of worldwide incomes. But its effect is most devastating on the individual level. Poor women and children are commodities traded on the street, products bartered, haggled over, smuggled, and sold as hedges against hunger or cruel-but-quick routes to profit.[57]

For example, consider the following:

- A seven-mile stretch of E55, a Czech motorway near the German border, is known as the "Highway of Cheap Love." E55 may be the longest brothel in the world, and on Saturday nights hundreds of Czech, German, Rumanian, Bulgarian, and Hungarian women, some as young as 15, line its shoulders to bargain with motorists—$30 for 30 minutes in the cab of a truck or a rundown motel.[58]

- Most Thai men have their first sexual encounter with one of the more than 2,000,000 prostitutes who work in that nation's thousands of brothels, massage parlors, coffee shops, and other fronts for the sex trade. A segment of Thailand's economy is dependent on the sex clubs and package sex tours that cater to international visitors.[59]

- In the brothels of Manila and Bangkok, the port sectors of Rio de Janeiro and Santos in Brazil, and the redlight districts of Eastern and Western Europe, pimps hawk the services of children as young as 8 years old—emphasizing that the children are "clean." It would appear that customers are willing to pay far more for very young boys and girls who are described as "virgins" or whose youth suggests innocence for a variety of reasons, including attempts to avoid contact with HIV. But this may be a mistaken belief, since both boys and girls are more vulnerable to infection because they are prone to lesions and injuries during anal and vaginal intercourse.[60]

- In Nepal's Himalayan villages, thousands of adolescents are sold each year to slave traders for the sweat-drenched brothels of Bombay; in Brazil an estimated 25,000 young girls have been forced into prostitution in remote Amazon mining camps; in Bologna, Nigerian streetwalkers are commonplace; and around Miami, massage parlors import prostitutes from Nicaragua, Colombia, and Canada.[61]

Within the context of these examples, the links between prostitution and AIDS, the bridging phenomenon involving prostitution and injection drug use, and the potential for the rapid heterosexual spread of the disease is gravely illustrated through the experience in Thailand. HIV was relatively late in arriving in Thailand (and other parts of Asia as well), so much so that in the early 1980s some Asian observers were suggesting that they had a natural immunity to the disease. The first reported case of AIDS in Thailand came in 1984, the patient was a homosexual man who had spent many years in the United States.[62] This, no doubt, was reassuring to many, for it fostered the notion that AIDS was going to be a disease of *farangs* (foreigners)—gay men and intravenous drug users. In fact, the disease spread quite slowly at first: between 1979 and 1986 the World Health Organization reported only six confirmed cases of AIDS in all of Thailand, six more cases in 1987, and none during the first half of 1988.[63] But ignored by Asian observers were some important factors—Thailand's international position in the production of opium and heroin, and its legions of intravenous drug use and commercial sex workers.

To begin with, a focal point in the trafficking complex of opium and heroin is the Golden Triangle, a vast area of Southeast Asia comprising the rugged Shan hills of Burma, the serpentine ridges of northern Thailand, and the upper highlands of Laos. This geographic area emerged during the late 1960s and early 1970s as the world's largest producer of illicit opium,[64] providing yields of some 700 metric tons annually. For a time, the Golden Triangle also dominated the heroin-refining markets of Western Europe, and there is considerable agreement that the growing of opium in the region was introduced by Chinese political refugees.

Using the Netherlands as their principal importation and distribution area, Chinese traffickers virtually controlled the heroin market—arranging for the purchase of raw opium, overseeing its conversion into heroin, and managing the international smuggling network. By 1978 to 1979, however, rivalries among the various Chinese drug syndicates, law-enforcement efforts against Asian traffickers, and declining production due to poor crop yields served to reduce the importance of the region as a center of opium trade.[65]

A second focal point in the opium-heroin trafficking complex is what has become known as the Golden Crescent, an arc of land stretching across Southwest Asia through sections of Pakistan, Iran, and Afghanistan. Emerging as the leading opium producer in the world during the late 1970s, the Golden Crescent successfully challenged its Southeast Asian counterpart by generating raw material for heroin that was less expensive and generally more potent. By the mid-1980s, over half the heroin entering the United States originated as opium in the Golden Crescent. Iran was the key opium producer, and Pakistan and Afghanistan were the primary heroin refiners and shippers, having numerous illicit laboratories on both sides of the Khyber Pass. By the close of the decade, however, with estimates suggesting that the combined yield of Southeast and Southwest Asian opium production exceeded 3,000 metric tons, the Golden Triangle had re-emerged as the world leader in opium production.[66]

But interestingly, in their efforts to regain control of the opium and heroin trade, early in the decade jungle laboratories began to appear in Thailand, Burma, and Laos, where the opium was refined into heroin and routed to the outside world by way of Bangkok. At the same time, when the increasing popularity of cocaine combined with a stabilizing population of narcotic addicts in the United States to reduce the demand for heroin, the Golden Triangle had bumper opium harvests, 600 tons annually—enough to make some 120 metric tons of heroin. The result was a surplus of the drug, at cheap prices, much of which found its way to the streets of Bangkok and other Thai cities. By the middle of the 1980s, at about the same time that the first cases of AIDS were being noticed, the number of intravenous heroin users in Thailand numbered in the hundreds of thousands.[67]

By 1987, a great majority of the Thai heroin injectors were sharing needles and other injection equipment, but the rates of HIV seropositivity remained relatively low. By 1988, however, the infection rate among injectors had increased to 15 percent, and during the next six months it soared to 43 percent.[68] In addition, more than a decade of official tourist materials depicting beautiful young women with "come hither" smiles had made Thailand's commercial sex industry notorious worldwide. The effort was attracting millions of tourists annually, the majority of whom were single men interested in sexual entertainment. Many of the prostitutes were heroin injectors, and by the early 1990s the proportion who were HIV-infected was estimated at 20 percent.[69] Importantly, sex with prostitutes is common among Thai men, and the World Health Organization has estimated that by the end of the 1990s as many as 4 million Thais will be HIV-infected, the majority of whom will be women.[70]

The nation that might repeat the Thai experience is Brazil, which currently has one of highest number of reported AIDS cases in the world, surpassed only by the United States and a few African countries. The first cases of AIDS in Brazil were identified in 1982 in the states of Rio de Janeiro and São Paulo, where one and four cases were recorded, respectively.[71] In 1983, 31 more cases were recognized, with substantial increases in subsequent years. By mid-1993, the total number of cases in Brazil exceeded 36,000,[72] with annual incidence rates per million population increasing from .05 in 1982 to 29.4 in 1990.[73]

The highest concentration of cases has occurred in the southeastern region of the country, which includes Rio de Janeiro and São Paulo, and among the 25- to 40-year-old age group. As is the case in the United States, homosexual/bisexual transmission accounts for the majority of cases, followed by heterosexual transmission and intravenous drug use. The actual number of AIDS cases in Brazil is likely grossly underestimated, given diagnostic deficiencies and the prevailing social climate.[74]

It would appear that any organized response to AIDS in Brazil has been minimal at best, likely the result of the perception at the beginning of the epidemic that it was a disease afflicting only wealthy homosexuals.[75] In addition, and more importantly, there is Brazil's precarious economic situation, its weak health-care system, and its inability to deal effectively with a whole array of parasitic, infectious, and other diseases, including malaria, typhoid, leprosy, schistosomiasis (from a waterborne parasite and resulting in intestinal bleeding, severe dysentery, and kidney failure) and *Trypanosoma cruzi* (another parasitic infection that ultimately results in congestive heart failure, and for which there is no known cure)—all of which are far more common and visible than HIV and AIDS.[76] Perhaps the largest factor in Brazil's failure to address the spread of AIDS is its depressed economic state, brought about by a foreign debt of over $115 billion. In this regard, for years Brazilians have been experiencing triple-digit inflation and the devaluation of their currency at a rate of 1 percent per day.

Within this context, for the better part of the 1980s the image of AIDS in Brazilian popular culture was that of a rare disease afflicting pockets of wealthy individuals who divided their time between Rio de Janeiro or São Paulo and such foreign cities as New York and Paris. Furthermore, AIDS patients were almost uniformly identified as highly promiscuous homosexual males.[77] By contrast, however, it would appear that HIV and AIDS in Brazil cut across all class, status, and income boundaries, having their greatest toll on lower-middle and lower class groups.[78] As in other societies, it is through sexual exchanges and contact with infected blood that the transmission of HIV takes place. As such, it is important to understand how these phenomena are socially and culturally constituted.

Although discussions of AIDS are typically considered under such groupings as "homosexuality," "bisexuality," and "heterosexuality," these categories are, in fact, highly problematic within the context of Brazilian sexual culture. More important are the notions of "atividade" (activity) and "passividade" (passivity) in sexual unions.[79] Brazilian males who are the so-called "active" partners in same-sex interactions, for example, do not necessarily consider themselves to be either "homosexual" or "bisexual." However, such labels *are* often reserved for the "passive" partners in these interactions. Moreover, not only is there negotiation of active and passive roles, but in addition, they do not preclude sexual interactions with the opposite sex. In short, while *sexual roles* (like partners) may vary, they tend to be far more significant than *sexual object choice* in the construction of one's sexual identity.[80] Moreover, occasional same-sex sexual relations are relatively unproblematic in the construction of a person's sexual identity.[81]

A product of this particular configuration of the sexual universe has been a certain fluidity in the formation of sexual relationships. These are ultimately reflected in the epidemiology of AIDS in Brazil and its unusually high level of transmission through "bisexual" contacts—19.5 percent.[82] Going further, what might be described as a sexual subculture based on same-sex interactions has somewhat flexible boundaries, organized more around same-sex desires than a shared "homosexual identity." For example, rather than the relative uniformity of a "gay subculture," in Brazil, there is a plurality of classifications and identities, including "miches" (hustlers), "travestis" (transvestites), effeminate "bichas" (literally "worms," but best translated as "queens"), self-consciously masculine "bofes" (studs), "sapatoes" ("dykes"), "sapatilhas" ("femme dykes"), and any number of other figures and variations.[83] Within the space of this subculture are scores of injection drug users, prostitutes, and considerable sexual intermingling. These factors, quite understandably, serve to accelerate the spread of HIV and AIDS among those at high risk in Brazil.

There are other issues as well. Importantly, members of this same-sex subculture also have relationships with the opposite sex.[84] Moreover, in heterosexual relationships both oral and anal sex take their place alongside vaginal intercourse as important elements in the cultural scripting of erotic interactions. At the same time, it is claimed that both married and unmarried men in Brazil use the services of prostitutes (from the sex clubs, brothels, *favelas* (shantytowns), and streets, including the homeless street youth) to engage in acts that "a proper wife and mother might shun."[85] Thus, of significance in Brazilian cities is not only the "primary spread" of HIV among those at highest risk, but also the "secondary spread" of HIV from those at high risk to other populations through heterosexual transmission.

POSTSCRIPT

In Africa, prostitutes are a main reservoir of sexually transmitted diseases.[86] Moreover, epidemiologic research has documented high rates of HIV infection among African prostitutes.[87] As a result of these and other studies, "promiscuity" per se has become a conventional explanation for the high rates of HIV infection in general, and heterosexual transmission of the virus in particular, in many African nations. However, since prostitution exists in virtually all societies and cultures, yet rates of heterosexual transmission of HIV vary markedly from one community to the next, better explanations are likely found in the social and cultural contexts of sexual and other behaviors and attitudes in any given society. Anthropological, sociological, and bio-behavioral studies in several parts of Africa have demonstrated this to be the case.

High rates of prostitution and sexually transmitted diseases do indeed exist in those parts of Africa most effected by the AIDS epidemic, but there are such additional factors as the frequency of polygyny, varying attitudes towards marriage and sexuality, sexual patterns involving small circles of interchanging lovers, and extensive migration between urban and rural areas.[88] Furthermore, in numerous cultures there are the following features: 1) practices resulting in exposure to blood, such as medicinal bloodletting, rituals establishing "blood brotherhood," and ritual and medicinal enemas; 2) practices involving the use of shared instruments, such as the injection of medicines, ritual scarification, group circumcision, genital tattooing, and the shaving of body hair; and 3) female "circumcision" and infibulation.*[89]

---

*Female circumcision is actually a euphemism for female genital mutilation. The most extreme, termed infibulation, involves partial closure of the vaginal orifice after excision of varying amounts of tissue from the vulva. Sometimes all of the mons veneris, labia majora and minora, and clitoris are removed and the involved areas are closed by means

In the United States, practices affecting the heterosexual spread of HIV can be illustrated through the experience in Belle Glade, Florida.[90] While early AIDS reports focused attention on gay and bisexual men and injection drug users in such large urban areas as San Francisco and New York City, the highest cumulative incidence rate of AIDS in the United States was being reported elsewhere—in a small rural sector of western Palm Beach County, Florida, an area that had an estimated population of some 29,000. While only 31 cases of AIDS had been reported in the area through 1985, in each subsequent year the number increased dramatically.

Belle Glade is a small farming town situated on the southeastern tip of Lake Okeechobee, in the heart of Florida's vegetable and sugar cane region. The permanent population of Belle Glade is supplemented by migrant workers who winter in the area, picking vegetables and citrus fruits. The population is also increased by sugar cane workers, predominantly from the Caribbean islands, who work the fields south of Belle Glade from November through March. In 1985, the per capita income in Belle Glade was $7,704, with more than 25 percent of the population living below the poverty level.[91] The incidence of disease in general, and sexually transmitted diseases in particular, is extremely high relative to the size of the population.[92]

In 1985, Belle Glade achieved national prominence when researchers at Miami's Institute of Tropical Medicine attributed the high rates of AIDS in Belle Glade to squalid living conditions and exposure to mosquitoes and other insects that encouraged infections that could trigger a dormant AIDS virus.[93] However, transmission by insect vectors, especially mosquitoes, has since been ruled out, as has the possible relationship between HIV and African swine fever virus.[94] In 1986, a Centers for Disease Control field study group evaluated the high cumulative incidence of AIDS through case interviews and neighborhood-based sero-epidemiologic studies.[95] The consensus of the scientific community to date has been that AIDS is spread in Belle Glade by the same mechanisms as elsewhere, namely through sexual contact and injection drug use.

Nevertheless, the epidemiology of the spread of AIDS in this small Florida community differs substantially from the national pattern, as well as from that seen in the state as a whole. While injection drug use has been considered a key factor, subsequent field studies in Belle Glade have demonstrated that there are actually few drug injectors in the area. Rather, the crucial element seems to be that the drug trade in Belle Glade is integrally associated with the sex industry—sex-for-

---

of sutures or thorns. More moderate forms of female circumcision involve the removal of the clitoris or the clitoral prepuce.

crack exchanges as discussed earlier in this chapter. One informant reported to the authors:

> I smoke so much rock, I don't care about how I look, I don't change my clothes or bathe, I have sex with anyone, I don't even look at them, I just want the rock.

Another stated:

> Everyone knows how you get AIDS, but the crack takes away your reason.

The rapid growth of the epidemic and the increasing percentage of heterosexually transmitted AIDS cases in Belle Glade suggest that the diffusion of HIV infection resembles that found in Pattern II countries—where the primary mode of transmission is heterosexual exposure and the ratio of male-to-female cases is almost 1-to-1.

What all of this suggests is that AIDS prevention and intervention efforts must be dynamic. In any given locale, these efforts must address specific community circumstances and contingencies, cultural differences, perceptions of vulnerability, and the social roles of those at risk.

END NOTES

1. Fintan R. Steele, "A Moving Target: CDC Still Trying to Estimate HIV-1 Prevalence," *Journal of NIH Research*, 6 (June 1994), p. 25

2. M. A. Fischl, G. M. Dickenson, G. B. Scott, N. Klimas, M. A. Fletcher, and W. Parks, "Evaluation of Heterosexual Partners, Children, and Household Contacts of Adults With AIDS," *Journal of the American Medical Association*, 257 (1987), pp. 640–644.

3. M. W. Vogt, D. E. Craven, D. Crawford, D. J. Witt, R. Byington, R. T. Schooley, and M. S. Hirsch, "Isolation of HTLV-III/LAV From Cervical Secretions of Women at Risk for AIDS," *Lancet* i (1986), pp. 525–527; M. W. Vogt, D. J. Witt, D. Craven, R. Byington, D. Crawford, M. S. Hutchinson, R. T. Schooley, and M. S. Hirsch, "Isolation Patterns of the Human Immunodeficiency Virus From Cervical Secretions During the Menstrual Cycle of Women at Risk for the Acquired Immunodeficiency Syndrome," *Annals of Internal Medicine*, 106 (1987), pp. 380–382; C. B. Wofsy, J. B. Cohen, L. B. Hauer, N. Padian, B. Michaelis, J. Evans, and J. A. Levy, "Isolation of AIDS-Associated Retrovirus from Genital Secretions of Women With Antibodies to the Virus,"*Lancet* i (1986), pp. 527–529.

4. R. A. Kasalow and D. P. Francis (eds.), *The Epidemiology of AIDS: Expression, Occurrence, and Control of Human Immunodeficiency Virus Type 1 Infection* (New York: Oxford University Press, 1989); P. Ma and D. Armstrong (eds.), *AIDS and Infections of Homosexual Men* (Boston: Butterworths, 1989).

5. A. M. Johnson, "Heterosexual Transmission of Human Immunodeficiency Virus," *British Medical Journal*, 296 (1988), pp. 1017–1020; European Study Group, "Risk Factors for Male to Female Transmission of HIV,"*British Medical Journal*, 298 (1989), pp. 411–415.

6. N. Hearst and B. H. Stephen, "Preventing the Heterosexual Spread of AIDS: Are We Giving Our Patients the Best Advice?" *Journal of the American Medical Association*, 259 (1988), pp. 24–28–2432; S. D. Holmberg, C. R. Horsburg, J. W. Ward, and H. W. Jaffe, "Biological Factors in the Heterosexual Transmission of Human Immunodeficiency Virus," *Journal of Infectious diseases*, 160 (1989), pp. 116–125.

7. N. Padian, J. Wiley, S. Glass, L. Marquis, and W. Winkelstein, "Anomalies of Infectivity in the Heterosexual Transmission of HIV," *IV International Conference on AIDS*, Stockholm, Sweden, June 12–18, 1988.

8. A. M. Johnson and M. Laga, "Heterosexual Transmission of HIV," *AIDS*, 2 (1988), Sup. 1), pp. S49–S56.

9. T. A. Peterman, R. L. Stoneburner, J. R. Allen, H. W. Jaffe, and J. W. Curran, "Risk of Human Immunodeficiency Transmission From Heterosexual Adults With Transfusion Associated Infections," *Journal of the American Medical Association*, 259 (1988), pp. 55–58; A. Johnson, A. Petherick, S. Davison, S. Howard, L. Osborne, C. Sonnex, R. Robertson, S. Tchamouroff, M. Hooker, R. Brettle, and M. W. Adler, "Transmission of HIV to Heterosexual Partners of Infected Men and Women," *IV International Conference on AIDS*, Stockholm, Sweden, June 12–18, 1988; M. Laga, H. Taelman, L. Bonneux, P. Cornet, G. Vercauteren, and P. Piot, "Risk Factors for Heterosexual Partners of HIV-Infected Africans and Europeans," *IV International Conference on AIDS*, Stockholm, Sweden,

June 12–18, 1988; J. J Goedert, M. E. Eyster, M. V. Ragni, R. J. Biggar, and M. H. Gail, "Rate of Heterosexual Transmission and Associated Risk with HIV Antigen," *IV International Conference on AIDS*, Stockholm, Sweden, 12-18 June 1988.

10. N. S. Padian, S. C. Shiboski, and N. P. Jewell, "The Effect of Number of Exposures on the Risk of Heterosexual HIV Transmission," *Journal of Infectious Diseases*, 161 (1990), pp. 883–887.

11. Marie Laga, Henri Taelman, Patrick Van der Stuyft, Luc Bonneux, Gaby Vercauteren, and Peter Piot, "Advanced Immunodeficiency as a Risk Factor for Heterosexual Transmission of HIV," *AIDS*, 3 (1989), pp. 361–366.

12. Adriano Lazzarin, Alberto Saracco, Massimo Musicco, and Alfredo Nicolosi, "Man–to–Woman Sexual Transmission of the Human Immunodeficiency Virus: Risk Factors Related to Sexual Behavior, Man's Infectiousness, and Woman's Susceptibility," *Annals of Internal Medicine*, 151 (1991), pp. 2411–2416.

13. N. Clumeck, M. Robert-Guroff, P. Van de Perre, A. Jennings, J. Sibomana, P. De Mol, S. Cran, and R. C. Gallo, "Seroepidemiological Studies of HTLV-III Antibody Prevalence Among Selected Groups of Heterosexual Africans, *Journal of the American Medical Association*, 254 (1985), p. 2599; D. W. Cameron, F. A. Plummer, and J. N. Simonsen, "Female to Male Heterosexual Transmission of HIV Infection in Nairobi," *III International Conference on AIDS*, Washington, DC, June 1–5, 1987; J. W. Carswell, G. Lloyd, and J. Howells, "Prevalence of HIV-1 in East African Lorry Drivers," *AIDS*, 3 (1989), pp. 759–761; J. K. Kreiss, D. Koech, and F. A. Plummer, "AIDS Virus Infection in Nairobi Prostitutes: Spread of the Epidemic in East Africa," *New England Journal of Medicine*, 314 (1986), p. 414.

14. J. L'Age-Stehr, A. Schwarz, and G. Offermann, "HTLV-III Infection in Kidney Transplant Recipients," *Lancet*, ii (1985), pp. 1361–1362.

15. L. H. Calabrese and K. V. Gopalakrishna, "Transmission of HTLV-III Infection From Man to Woman to Man," *New England Journal of Medicine*, 314 (1986), p. 987.

16. T. Barnett and P. Blaikie, *AIDS in Africa: Its Present and Future Impact* (New York: Guilford Press, 1992); Panos Institute, *AIDS and the Third World* (London: Panos Publications, 1988); G. W. Shannon, G. F. Pyle, and R. I. Bashshur, *The Geography of AIDS: Origins and Course of the Epidemic* (New York: Guilford Press, 1991).

17. E. J. Beck, C. Donegan, C. S. Cohen, C. Kenny, V. Moss, G.S. Underhill, P. Terry, D. J. Jeffries, A. J. Pinching, D. L. Miller, D. G. Cunningham, and J. R. W. Harris, "Risk Factors for HIV-1 Infection in a British Population: Lessons From a London Sexually Transmitted Disease Clinic," *AIDS*, 3 (1989), pp. 533–538; European Study Group, "Comparison of Female to Male and Male to Female Transmission of HIV in 563 Stable Couples," *British Medical Journal*, 304 (1992), pp. 809–813; A. M. Johnson, A. Petherick, S. J. Davidson, R. Brettle, M. Hooker, L. Howard, K. A. McLean, L. E. M. Osborne, R. Robertson, C. Sonnex, S. Tchamouroff, C. Shergold, and M. W. Adler, "Transmission of HIV to Heterosexual Partners of Infected Men and Women," *AIDS*, 3 (1989), pp. 367–372; J. J. Lefrere, D. Vittecoq, M. L. North, W. Smilovici, P. Aubertin, M. Gueguen, A. Nicod, T. Lambert, and C. Janot, "Risk of Female to Male Transmission of HIV From Women Infected by Transfusion," *AIDS*, 2 (1988), pp. 137–138.

18. G. H. Friedland and R. S. Klein, "Transmission of Human Immunodeficiency Virus," *New England Journal of Medicine*, 317 (1987), pp. 1125–1135; D. Osmond, "Heterosexual Transmission of HIV," in P. T. Cohen, M. A. Sande, and P. A. Volberding (eds.), *The AIDS Knowledge Base* (Waltham, MA: Massachusetts Medical Society, 1990), pp. 1.2.4:1–9.

19. D. S. Burke and R. R. Redfield, "Transmission of Human Immunodeficiency Virus (HIV)," *New England Journal of Medicine*, 318 (1988), pp. 1202–1203.

20. Harry W. Haverkos and Robert J. Battjes, "Female-to-Male Transmission of HIV," *Journal of the American Medical Association*, 268 (1992), p. 1855.

21. J. B. Cohen, P. Alexander, and C. Wofsy, "Prostitutes and AIDS: Public Policy Issues," *AIDS and Public Policy Journal*, 3 (1988), pp. 16–22.

22. J. B. Cohen, "Sexual Transmission Associated With Commercial Sex," *National Institute on Drug Abuse AIDS Research Planning Meeting*, Rockville, MD, 23-24 Jan. 1992.

23. Carswell et al. 1989; Shannon et al. 1991; Barnett and Blaikie 1992.

24. J. N. Simonsen, D. W. Cameron, M. N. Gakinya, J. O. Ndinya-Achola, L. J. D'Costa, P. Karasira, M. Cheang, A. R. Ronald, P. Piot, and F. A. Plummer, "Human Immunodeficiency Virus Infection Among Men With Sexually Transmitted Diseases," *New England Journal of Medicine*, 319 (1988), pp. 274–278; D. W. Cameron, L. J. D'Costa, G. M. Maitha, M. Cheang, P. Piot, J. N. Simonsen, A. R. Ronald, M. N. Gakinya, J. O. Ndinya-Achola, R. C. Brunham, and F. A. Plummer, "Female to Male Transmission of Human Immunodeficiency Virus Type 1: Risk Factors for Seroconversion in Men," *Lancet*, ii (1989), pp. 403–407; N. O'Farrell, "Transmission of HIV: Genital Ulceration, Sexual Behavior, and Circumcision," *Lancet*, ii (1989), p. 1157; P. Piot, J. K. Kreiss, J. O. Ndinya-Achola, E. N. Ngugi, J. N. Simonsen, D. W. Cameron, H. Tealman, and F. A. Plummer, "Editorial Review: Heterosexual Transmission of HIV," *AIDS*, 1 (1987), pp. 199–206; F. A. Plummer, J. N. Simonsen, D. W. Cameron, J. O. Ndinya-Achola, J. K. Kreiss, M. N. Gakinya, P. Waiyaki, M. Cheang, P. Piot, A. R. Ronald, and E. N. Ngugi, "Cofactors in Male–Female Sexual Transmission of Human Immunodeficiency Virus Type 1," *Journal of Infectious Diseases*. 163 (1991), pp. 233–239.

25. See Cohen, 1992.

26. A. Carmen and H. Moody, *Working Women: The Subterranean World of Street Prostitution* (New York: Harper & Row, 1985); H. Evans, *Harlots, Whores and Hookers: A History of Prostitution* (New York: Dorset Books, 1979); Paul J. Goldstein, *Prostitution and Drugs* (Lexington, MA: Lexington Books, 1979); B. S. Heyl, *The Madam as Entrepreneur: Career Management in House Prostitution* (New Brunswick, NJ: Transaction Books, 1979); E. M. Miller, *Street Women* (Philadelphia: Temple University Press, 1986); Marsha Rosenbaum, *Women on Heroin* (New Brunswick, NJ: Rutgers University Press, 1981); Charles Winick and P. M. Kinsie, *The Lively Commerce: Prostitution in the United States* (Chicago: Quadrangle Books, 1971).

27. Heyl, 1979.

28. J. Gross, "A New, Purified Form of Cocaine Causes Alarm as Abuse Increases," *The New York Times*, 29 Nov. 1985, pp. 1A, B6; J. V. Lamar,

"Crack," *Time*, 2 June 1986, pp. 16–18; J. Lawlor, "USA Battles Souped-Up Cocaine," *USA Today*, 16 June 1986, pp. 1A–2A.

29. James A. Inciardi, "Trading Sex for Crack Among Juvenile Drug Users: A Research Note," *Contemporary Drug Problems*, 16 (1989), pp. 689–700.

30. Benjamin Bowser, "Crack and AIDS: An Ethnographic Impression," *Journal of the National Medical Association*, 81 (1989), pp. 538–540; Mindy Thompson Fullilove and Robert E. Fullilove, "Intersecting Epidemics: Black Teen Crack Use and Sexually Transmitted Disease," *Journal of the American Women's Medical Association*, 44 (1989), pp. 146–153; Robert E. Fullilove, Mindy Thompson Fullilove, Benjamin B. Bowser, and S. A. Gross, "Risk of Sexually Transmitted Disease Among Black Adolescent Crack Users in Oakland and San Francisco, California," *Journal of the American Medical Association*, 263 (1990), pp. 851–855; P. Kerr, "Crack and Resurgence of Syphilis Spreading AIDS Among the Poor," *The New York Times*, 20 Aug. 1989, p. 1; A. Knopf, "Syphilis and Crack Linked in Connecticut," *Substance Abuse Report*, 1 Aug. 1989, pp. 1–2; A. Knopf, "Syphilis and Gonorrhea on the Rise Among Inner-City Drug Addicts," *Substance Abuse Report*, 1 June 1989, pp. 1–2.

31. M. A. Chiasson, R. L. Stoneburner, D. S. Hildebrandt, W. E. Ewing, E. E. Telzak, and H. W. Jaffee, "Heterosexual Transmission of HIV-1 Associated With the Use of Smokable Freebase Cocaine (Crack)," *AIDS*, 5 (1991), pp. 1121–1126.

32. D. C. Des Jarlais, A. Abdul-Quader, H. Minkoff, B. Hoegsberg, S. Landesman, and S. Tross, "Crack Use and Multiple AIDS Risk Behaviors," *Journal of Acquired Immune Deficiency Syndromes*, 4 (1991), pp. 446–447.

33. Mitchell S. Ratner (ed.), *Crack Pipe as Pimp: An Ethnographic Investigation of Sex-for-Crack Exchanges* (New York: Lexington Books, 1993).

34. See H. Virginia McCoy, Christine Miles, and James A. Inciardi, "Survival Sex: Inner-City Women and Crack-Cocaine," in James A. Inciardi and Karen McElrath (eds.), *The American Drug Scene* (Los Angeles: Roxbury Publishing Co., 1995).

35. Lester Grinspoon and James B. Bakalar, *Cocaine: A Drug and Its Social Evolution* (New York: Basic Books, 1976); Roger D. Weiss and Steven M. Mirin, *Cocaine* (Washington, DC: American Psychiatric Press, 1987).

36. James A. Inciardi, Dorothy Lockwood, and Anne E. Pottieger, *Women and Crack-Cocaine* (New York: Macmillan, 1993); Ratner, 1993.

37. John C. Ball and Carl D. Chambers, *The Epidemiology of Opiate Addiction in the United States* (Springfield, IL: Charles C. Thomas, 1970); Rosenbaum, 1981.

38. Inciardi, Lockwood, and Pottieger.

39. H. Virginia McCoy and Christine Miles, "A Gender Comparison of Health Status Among Users of Crack Cocaine," *Journal of Psychoactive Drugs*, 24 (1992), pp. 389–397; Ratner; Inciardi, Lockwood, and Pottieger.

40. Inciardi, Lockwood, and Pottieger.

41. James A. Inciardi, Dale D. Chitwood, and Clyde B. McCoy, "Special Risks for the Acquisition and Transmission of HIV Infection During Sex in Crack Houses," *Journal of Acquired Immune Deficiency Syndromes*, 5 (1992), pp. 951–952.

42. J. R. Magana, "Sex, Drugs, and HIV: An Ethnographic Investigation," *Social Science and Medicine*, 33 (1991), pp. 5–9.

43. M. A. Fischl, "Prevention of Transmission of AIDS During Sexual Inter-course, in V. T. DeVita, S. Hellman, and S. A. Rosenberg (eds.), *AIDS: Etiology, Diagnosis, Treatment, and Prevention* (Philadelphia: J.B. Lippin-cott, 1988), pp. 369–374; V. Puro, N. Narciso, E. Girardi, L. Antonelli, M. Zaccarelli, and G. Visco, "Male-to-Female Transmission of Human Immu-nodeficiency Virus Infection by Oro-Genital Sex," *European Journal of Clinical Microbiology and Infectious Diseases*, 10 (1991), p. 47.

44. I. P. M. Keet, N. A. van Lent, T. G. M. Sandfort, R. A. Coutinho, and G. J. P. van Griensven, "Orogenital Sex and the Transmission of HIV Among Homosexual Men," *AIDS*, 6 (1992), pp. 223–226; A. R. Lifson, P. M. O'Mal-ley, N. A. Hessol, S. P. Buchbinder, L. Cannon, and G. W. Rutherford, "HIV Seroconversion in Two Homosexual Men After Receptive Oral In-tercourse With Ejaculation: Implications for Counseling Concerning Safe Sexual Practices," *American Journal of Public Health*, 80 (1990), pp. 1509–1511; W. Rozenbaum, S. Gharakhanian, B. Cardon, E. Duval, and J. P. Coulaud, "HIV Transmission by Oral Sex," *Lancet*, i (1988), p. 1395.

45. P. G. Spitzer and N. J. Weiner, "Transmission of HIV Infection From a Woman to a Man by Oral Sex," *New England Journal of Medicine*, 320 (1989), p. 251.

46. Centers for Disease Control, "Acquired Immunodeficiency Syndrome (AIDS)—United States," *Morbidity and Mortality Weekly Report*, 33 (1984), p. 661.

47. Harry W. Haverkos and Robert Edelman, "Female-to-Male Transmission of AIDS," *Journal of the American Medical Association*, 254 (1985), pp. 1035–1036.

48. B. Frank Polk, "Female-to-Male Transmission of AIDS," *Journal of the American Medical Association*, 254 (1985), pp. 3177–3178.

49. Erik Eckholm, "Prostitutes' Impact on Spread of AIDS Is Debated," *The New York Times*, 5 Nov. 1985, pp. C1, C8.

50. Philippe Van de Perre, Nathan Clumeck, Michel Careal, Elie Nzabihi-mana, Marjorie Robert-Guroff, Patrick De Mol, Pierre Freyens, Jean-Paul Butzler, Robert C. Gallo, and Jean-Baptiste Kanyamupira, "Female Pros-titutes: A Risk Group for Infection With Human T-Cell Lymphotropic Virus Type III," *Lancet*, ii (1985), pp. 524–526.

51. See Barbara C. Leigh, Mark T. Temple, and Karen F. Trocki, "The Sexual Behavior of U.S. Adults: Results From a National Survey," *American Jour-nal of Public Health*, 83 (1993), pp. 1400–1408.

52. John O. G. Billy, Koray Tanfer, William R. Grady, and Daniel H. Klepinger, "The Sexual Behavior of Men in the United States," *Family Planning Per-spectives*, 25 (1993), pp. 52–60.

53. Mindell Seidlin, Keith Krasinski, Donna Bebenroth, Vincenza Itri, Anna Maira Paolino, and Fred Valentine, "Prevalence of HIV Infection in New York Call Girls," *Journal of Acquired Immune Deficiency Syndromes*, 1 (1988), pp. 150–154.

54. Joyce Wallace, "AIDS in Prostitutes," in Pearl Ma and Donald Armstrong (eds.), *AIDS and Infections of Homosexual Men* (Boston: Butterworths, 1989), pp. 285–295.

55. See William W. Sanger, *The History of Prostitution: Its Extent, Causes and Effects Throughout the World* (New York: Medical Publishing Co., 1899); Fernando Henriques, *Prostitution in Europe and the Americas* (New York: Citadel Press, 1965).

56. Edgar Gregersen, *Sexual Practices: The Story of Human Sexuality* (New York: Franklin Watts, 1983), pp. 149–166.

57. Margot Hornblower, "The Skin Trade," *Time*, 21 June 1993, pp. 45–51.

58. Hornblower, p. 45.

59. Ken Stier, "Waking Up to a Death Threat," *Los Angeles Times*, 17 May 1993, p. B6.

60. Bruce Crumley, Ann M. Simmons, and Rhea Schoenthal, "Defiling the Children," *Time*, 21 June 1993, pp. 52–55; Marlise Simons, "The Sex Market: Scourge of the World's Children," *The New York Times*, 9 April 1993, p. A3.

61. Neil McKenna, "A Disaster Waiting to Happen," *WorldAIDS*, May 1993, pp. 5–9; Margot Hornblower, "The Skin Trade," *Time*, 21 June 1993, pp. 45–51.

62. *AIDS and the Third World* (London: Panos Institute, 1988), p. 29.

63. World Health Organization, "Update: AIDS Cases Reported to Surveillance, Forecasting, and Impact Assessment Unit, Global Program on AIDS, 30 June 1988.

64. See Alfred W. McCoy, *The Politics of Heroin in Southeast Asia* (New York: Harper & Row, 1972); Editors of Newsday, *The Heroin Trail* (New York: New American Library, 1974); Jon A. Wiant, "Narcotics in the Golden Triangle," *Washington Quarterly*, 8 (Fall 1985), pp. 125–140.

65. For an examination of the hill tribes that populate the Golden Triangle and how opium cultivation impacts on their culture, see Paul Lewis and Elaine Lewis, *Peoples of the Golden Triangle: Six Tribes in Thailand* (London: Thames and Hudson, 1984); Claudia Simms and Thomas Tarleton, "The Lisu of the Golden Triangle," *The World & I*, October 1987, pp. 461–473.

66. Bureau of International Narcotics Matters, *International Narcotics Control Strategy Report* (Washington, DC: Department of State, March 1990), p. 18.

67. James A. Inciardi, *The War on Drugs: Heroin, Cocaine, Crime, and Public Policy* (Palo Alto, CA: Mayfield, 1986), p. 193.

68. Peter Gould, *The Slow Plague: A Geography of the AIDS Pandemic* (Oxford: Blackwell, 1993), p. 92.

69. Ron Moreau, "Sex and Death in Thailand, " *Newsweek*, 20 July 1992, p. 50.

70. Moreau.

71. L. Rodrigues and P. Chequer, "AIDS in Brazil, 1982–1988," *PAHO Bulletin*, 23 (1989), pp. 30–34.

72. World Health Organization, "Acquired Immunodeficiency Syndrome (AIDS) Data as of 30 June 1993," *Weekly Epidemiological Record*, 68 (2 July 1993).

73. Pan American Health Organization, *AIDS Surveillance in the Americas*, PAHO/WHO Global Program on AIDS, 16 September 1991.

74. T. C. Quinn, J. P. Narain, and R. K. Zacarais, "AIDS in the Americas: A Public Health Priority for the Region," *AIDS*, 4 (1990), pp. 709–724.

75. Richard G. Parker, "Responding to AIDS in Brazil," in B. A. Misztal and D. Moss (eds.), *Action on AIDS: National Policies in Comparative Perspective* (Westport, CT: Greenwood Press, 1990), pp. 52–77.

76. Paul F. Basch, *Textbook of International Health* (New York: Oxford, 1990); J. Lang, *Inside Development in Latin America: A Report from the Dominican Republic, Colombia, and Brazil* (Chapel Hill: University of North Carolina Press, 1988).

77. H. Daniel, "A Sindrome do Preconceito," *Comunicacoes do ISER*, 4 (1985), pp. 48–56; J. Galvao, "AIDS: A 'Doenca' e os 'Doentes'," *Comunicacoes do ISER*, 4 (1985), pp. 42–47.

78. C. D. Guimaraes, "A Questao dos Preconceitos," *ABIA: Boletim*, 3 (1988), pp. 2–3.

79. Richard G. Parker, "Acquired Immunodeficiency Syndrome in Urban Brazil," *Medical Anthropology Quarterly*, 1 (1987), pp. 155–175.

80. Richard G. Parker, "Youth, Identity and Homosexuality: The Changing Shape of Sexual Life in Contemporary Brazil," *Journal of Homosexuality*, 17 (1989), pp. 137–163.

81. P. Fry, *Para Ingles Ver: Identidade a Politica na Cultura Brasileira* (Rio de Janeiro: Zahar Editores, 1982); Richard G. Parker, "Masculinity, Femininity, and Homosexuality: On the Anthropological Interpretation of Sexual Meanings in Brazil," *Journal of Homosexuality*, 11 (1985), pp. 155–163.

82. Pan American Health Organization.

83. Richard G. Parker, *Bodies, Pleasures and Passions: Sexual Culture in Contemporary Brazil* (Boston: Beacon Press, 1991).

84. P. Fry, "Male Homosexuality and the Spirit of Possession in Brazil," *Journal of Homosexuality*, 11 (1985), pp. 137–153.

85. R. Freitas, *Bordel, Bordeis: Negociando Identidades* (Petropolis: Editora Vozes Ltda., 1985).

86. Lourdes J. D'Costa, Francis A. Plummer, Ian Bowmer, Lieve Fransen, Peter Piot, Allan R. Ronald, and Herbert Nsanze, "Prostitutes are a Major Reservoir of Sexually Transmitted Diseases in Nairobi, Kenya," *Sexually Transmitted Diseases*, 12 (1985), pp. 64–67.

87. Joan J. Kreiss, Davy Koech, Francis A. Plummer, King K. Holmes, Marilyn Lightfoote, Peter Piot, Allan R. Ronald, J. O. Ndinya-Achola, Lourdes J. D'Costa, Pacita Roberts, Elizabeth N. Ngugi, and Thomas C. Quinn, "AIDS Virus Infection in Nairobi Prostitutes: Spread of the Epidemic to East Africa," *New England Journal of Medicine*, 314 (1986), pp. 414–418; Nzilambi Nzila, Marie Laga, Manoka Abib Thiam, Kivuvu Mayimona, B. Edidi, Eddy Van Dyck, Frieda Behets, Susan Hassig, Ann Nelson, K. Mokwa, Rhoda L. Ashley, Peter Piot, and Robert W. Ryder, "HIV and Other Sexually Transmitted Diseases Among Female Prostitutes in Kinshasa," *AIDS*, 5 (1991), pp. 715–721.

88. See Ann Larson, "Social Context of Human Immunodeficiency Virus Transmission in Africa: Historical and Cultural Bases of East and Central African Sexual Relations," *Reviews of Infectious Diseases*, 11 (1989), pp. 716–731; Tony Barnett and Piers Blaikie, *AIDS in Africa: Its Present and Future Impact* (New York: Guilford Press, 1992).

89. See Daniel B. Hardy, "Cultrual Practices Contributing to the Transmission of Human Immunodeficiency Virus in Africa," *Reviews of Infectious Diseases*, 9 (1987), pp. 1109–1119; Meredeth Turshen (ed.), *Women and Health in Africa* (Trenton, NJ: Africa World Press, 1991).

90. See Dale D. Chitwood, James A. Inciardi, Duane C. McBride, Clyde B. McCoy, H. Virginia McCoy, and Edward Trapido, *A Community Approach to AIDS Intervention: Exploring the Miami Outreach Project for Injection Drug Users and Other High Risk Groups* (Westport, CT: Greenwood Press, 1991), pp. 123–130.

91. *Florida Statistical Abstract* (Gainesville: University of Florida, 1989).

92. Edward J. Trapido, Nancy Lewis and Mary Comerford, "HIV-1 and AIDS in Belle Glade, Florida: A Re-examination of the Issues," *American Behavioral Scientist*, 33 (1990), pp. 451–464.

93. K. Leishman, "AIDS and Insects," *Atlantic Monthly*, 260 (1987), pp. 56–72.

94. Colin Norman, "Sex and Needles, Not Insects and Pigs, Spread AIDS in Florida Town," *Science*, 234 (1986), pp. 415–417.

95. Kenneth G. Castro, Spencer Lieb, Harold W. Jaffe, John P. Narkunas, Charles H. Calisher, Timothy J. Bush, John J. Witte, and the Belle Glade Field Study Group, "Transmission of HIV in Belle Glade, Florida: Lessons for Other Communities in the United States," *Science*, 239 (1988), pp. 193–197.

CHAPTER FIVE

HIV/AIDS Prevention and Risk Reduction

The late American poet John Ciardi, perhaps best known for his translation of Dante Alighieri's *Inferno*, once commented that "all wives become Monday-morning quarterbacks by the tenth anniversary, although mine made that varsity in six months."[1] In this sexist wisecrack, Ciardi was referring to the "experts" who emerge *after the fact*. In contemporary English usage, the Monday-morning quarterback is the observer who calls the plays after the game, and who is, therefore, as infallibly right as hindsight makes anyone. Originally the expression was limited to football spectators,* but now it refers to anyone who is good at predicting things that have already happened and at pointing out the errors of any decision maker. As in the sports arena and in everyday life, the AIDS era has had its share of Monday-morning quarterbacks, with the majority focusing their attention on what *should* have been done when the epidemic first started.

A decade ago, even before the human immunodeficiency virus (HIV) was discovered to be the cause of AIDS, some virologists were confidently predicting that a vaccine was right around the corner, and that AIDS—like diabetes and asthma—would soon be considered a chronic, but treatable, ailment. However, it has not turned out that way. HIV is a clever and wily virus. Until recently, researchers were optimistic about a dozen or so vaccines under development. Using components of HIV grown in the laboratory, they hoped to design vaccines that would trick the immune system into producing effective antibodies.** When they injected these vaccines

---

*There was a time, many years ago, when all football games were played on Saturdays, allowing Monday-morning quarterbacks most of the weekend to sharpen their hindsights.

**As noted earlier in Chapter One, the presence of specific antibodies in the blood

into human volunteers, the immune systems did indeed make antibodies. These, in turn, seemed to block the HIV grown in the laboratory.
This is the way that all vaccines are developed. When tested against
HIV isolated from people, however, the antibodies failed. Apparently,
the virus mutates so rapidly that there are major differences between
wild and laboratory-grown HIV.[2]

These and other setbacks have provided a forum for the many Monday-morning quarterbacks and other kibitzers, jesters, provocateurs,
and gadflies who patrol the borders of scientific inquiry and policy-
making. Among the more visible of these has been Dr. Peter Duesberg,
a rather well-known virologist from the University of California at
Berkeley. Dr. Duesberg has claimed that HIV is *not* the cause of AIDS,[3]
despite the overwhelming evidence judging that it is and the concur-
rence of research virologists on several continents.[4] To "prove" his
point Duesberg even volunteered to drink a cup of HIV on national
television,[5] a rather hollow gesture since the virus would most likely be
killed by stomach acids before it could infect him.

There have been many other Monday-morning players and coaches,
emphasizing what *should* and *should not* have been done in terms of
funding, research, and policy. Yet not all instances of retrospective
deliberation and reflection are without value. In 1993, for example, Dr.
Martin Fishbein of the University of Illinois and a Guest Researcher at
the Centers for Disease Control and Prevention made the following
comments:

> In the early days of the epidemic, almost all support for AIDS research
> was directed at the medical and epidemiological communities. And, it
> wasn't until epidemiologists identified the modes of HIV transmission
> that it became clear to many that primary prevention was, first and
> foremost, a behavioral problem. Even with this recognition, support for
> behavioral research was slow in coming. Funding was and still is dis-
> proportionately directed at medical research.[6]

Similarly, the National Commission on AIDS concluded in 1993
that, to a very great extent, the potential contributions of behavioral
and social sciences have not been utilized in the battle against AIDS.[7]
In 1994, a panel of the National Academy of Sciences concluded, after
a thorough review of the AIDS research portfolio, that a lack of studies
on sexual behavior and drug use had blocked progress in fighting
AIDS.[8] The report by the 16-member committee also noted that the
basic research on how to try to change people's behavior had not been
done; that such basic research had been inhibited by a political climate

---

indicates that a previous infection registered on the body's immune system. The antibody
molecules that remain in the bloodstream act as scouts, so to speak: if the virus appears
again, the scouts recognize it immediately and attempt to prevent it from getting a
foothold.

during the first decade of the epidemic that made it difficult, and on some occasions impossible, to conduct the research on the very behaviors in question—drug use and sex.

What the behavioral and social sciences have to offer are approaches for designing and evaluating effective AIDS prevention initiatives. The point is this: in the absence of an effective vaccine or cure for AIDS, and while the virologists, biologists, and other medical researchers search for the elusive "magic bullet," the only alternatives are prevention, risk reduction, and behavioral change.

AIDS EDUCATION: SOME GENERAL CONSIDERATIONS

The great majority of early AIDS prevention/intervention programs were based on a general education model stressing increased awareness of, and knowledge about, the disease. Programs included education campaigns targeting the specific groups that were at the greatest risk of HIV acquisition and transmission—gay men and intravenous drug users. AIDS awareness programs also targeted the general population. In fact, in 1988, as part of the Department of Health and Human Services' nationwide public education program, the eight-page brochure *Understanding AIDS* was mailed to every household in the United States.[9] In all, 107 million English-language versions of the booklet were delivered (and a Spanish version was distributed in Puerto Rico), representing the first time in the history of the United States that the federal government attempted to contact virtually every resident, directly by mail, about a major public health problem.*

The effectiveness of public education programs has been questioned, however, in light of only minimal evidence suggesting that informational material correlates with risk reduction.[10] For example, one investigation found that while 85 percent of the participants in a risk-reduction effort agreed with the statement "the fewer sexual partners you have the less risk there is of getting the virus," their mean number of sexual partners actually increased during the course of the study.[11] Furthermore, while 70 percent of these respondents reported that they had never used a condom, 90 percent *disagreed* with the statement "the hassle of using a condom isn't worth the protection it gives." Similarly, studies of gay men have found that neither atten-

---

*Interestingly, it was alleged that the Reagan White House had delayed the dissemination of the report because it contained references to oral and anal sex. On July 31, 1987, Surgeon General C. Everett Koop met with White House staff, who requested the removal of the recommendation that condoms be used during sexual intercourse. The material on condoms remained in the brochure. See *AIDS Education: Printing and Distribution of the Surgeon General's Report* (Washington, D.C.: United States General Accounting Office, 1988).

dance at safe sex lectures, receiving advice from physicians about AIDS, getting an AIDS test, nor reading safe sex brochures are associated with participation in safe sex.[12]

There seem to be many reasons why the mere transfer of knowledge is typically insufficient to modify established behavior patterns. For example, people may understand and learn what public health professionals want them to know, but they may not consider the information to be personally relevant to them. They may not see themselves at risk, or they may not feel that they are capable of modifying the behaviors that place them at risk.

By contrast, risk-reduction programs that include informational messages coupled with group interactions and exercises seem to do better. For example, in an effort designed to reduce the frequency of sexual risk behaviors among black male adolescents, study subjects were randomly assigned to either an AIDS risk-reduction program or a career opportunities program.[13] The risk-reduction condition consisted of a five-hour intervention designed to increase the youths' knowledge of AIDS and sexually transmitted diseases, alter their attitudes toward risky sex, and provide information about the risks associated with injection drug use. A feature of the intervention was the use of interactive games and videos. Participants in the control condition were exposed to a five-hour career planning workshop that made use of videotapes, small group discussions, exercises, and games. They did not receive AIDS prevention information. At follow-up, the AIDS information condition participants reported engaging in fewer risky sexual behaviors than did the career opportunities youths. They reported having fewer sexual encounters overall, and particularly with women who were in sexual relationships with other men. They also reported more frequent use of condoms than those in the control condition.

It has been argued that behaviors are difficult to change when they are longstanding, highly and immediately reinforced, and when the threat of a negative health outcome is far removed in time from the behavior conferring the risk.[14] Within this context, a suggested risk reduction involves the redefinition of traditional peer group norms as socially unacceptable, with risk-reduction behaviors as more appropriate. This "reasoned action model" of behavioral change has been widely used in the gay community through discussion groups aimed at establishing group norms that promote healthy behavior. The STOP AIDS initiative, for example, established in San Francisco's gay community in 1984, uses this approach. Group discussions consist of conversations about the impact of AIDS on the participants' lives, modes of virus transmission through risky versus safe sex, the relationships between unsafe sex and drug and alcohol use, injection drug use and virus transmission, and HIV antibody testing. STOP AIDS sessions also include discussions about the changes taking place in the gay community as a result of the AIDS epidemic, and how each participant can be personally involved in ending the epidemic. Follow-up studies have found the STOP AIDS program to be effective in promoting risk-reduction behaviors.[15]

There are numerous varieties of risk-reduction programs, many of which are effective and others that are not particularly so. Some approaches involve literature and lectures on HIV-risk behaviors combined with skills and assertiveness training,[16] HIV testing and counseling,[17] audiovisual presentations and individual counseling,[18] or couple counseling in conjunction with social supports.[19] These and other intervention strategies are far from perfect, but they have been found to be considerably more effective than the simple, passive transfer of AIDS prevention information. The most effective interventions, furthermore, seem to be those that are culturally appropriate and designed for specific target populations, keeping in mind the attitudes, values, and concerns of those populations, including the social and economic barriers that may inhibit attempts at behavioral change. And perhaps most difficult to influence of all risk groups have been injection drug users and their sexual partners.

TARGETING INJECTION DRUG USERS

Injection drug users represent a group at risk for transmitting HIV infection not only to themselves but to non-injecting gays, heterosexuals, and perinatal cases. Sex with an injection drug user accounts for more than half of all reported AIDS cases through heterosexual contacts in the United States. Similarly, well over half of all reported pediatric AIDS cases have some association with injection drug use—involving mothers at risk of HIV infection through injecting drugs and/or through sex with an injector. There are estimates that 23 percent to 60 percent of the heterosexual partners of injection drug users, depending on the urban locale, have contracted HIV infection.[20] Transmission occurs most often from male to female, and the majority of those infected are non-injecting women.[21]

Many of the issues surrounding the spread of HIV infection to sex partners are rooted in subcultural issues of trust, since the lives of most injection users are beset with insecurity, apprehension, fragile relationships, and minimal kinship. As such, the kinds of behavioral changes appropriate for HIV risk reduction have the potential for introducing elements of suspicion into a relationship. It has been argued, for example, that to ask a sex partner to use a condom is in direct contradiction to the gender roles existing in the street drug culture.[22] More specifically, a woman's request of her man to use a condom not only compromises her prescribed role in the relationship, but also suggests that she believes her partner to be "contaminated" in some way. The reverse could also be the case when a male injection user begins using condoms with his partner.

Going further, the existence of shooting galleries across the urban landscape combined with the drug-taking and sexual behaviors of injection drug users pose a dilemma. Although most, if not virtually all, drug users are aware of AIDS and the risk of infection through unprotected sex and the multiple use of common injection equipment, in many instances the prevention messages are either not listened to or not followed. The problem is this: heroin and cocaine are highly seductive drugs. For those dependent on them, the drugs become life-consuming. They become mother, father, spouse, lover, counselor, confessor, and confidant. Since they are short-acting drugs, they must be taken regularly and repeatedly. Because there is a more rapid onset and a more powerful euphoric "high" when the drugs are taken intravenously, most heroin users and a growing number of cocaine users inject their drugs. Collectively, these attributes result in a majority of chronic users more concerned with drug-taking and drug-seeking than with careers, relationships, or health. As such, it would appear that altering the risk behaviors of drug users might be difficult. Or as one intravenous cocaine-using prostitute summed it up:

> Every day I risk my health, and my life for that matter, when I shoot up. Every time I go out to cop [buy drugs] I risk getting cut [stabbed] or even killed. Every time I'm strolling [walking the streets soliciting clients] at night, there are all kinds of crazies, geeks, thugs, and death freaks out there just waiting to carve up my ass. Now they say that if I use some dirty needle I can get sick, even die in a few years. So I care? I'm probably already dead. Why should I care?

In other words, it is difficult to prevent behavior that may cause sickness and death in two or five or more years when the injection drug user is confronted with violence, sickness, and death almost every day; it is difficult to motivate behaviors aimed at preventing death in the future within a population already at high risk of imminent death.

Within this context, only the most naïve would attempt to change the HIV-risk behaviors of drug injectors through simple AIDS prevention messages. Drug-using and sexual behaviors are learned and internalized practices, strengthened by time and repetition; and they may define a preferred lifestyle, be driven by physiological and/or psychological dependence, and be perceived by the persons involved as essential to the maintenance of valued personal and sexual relationships. From the more vital perspectives of societal values and their reflection in public policy, there is a prevalent perception that drug injectors, by their very "nature" and definition, are both self-destructive and incapable of sustaining long-term behavioral changes. However, a number of studies provide accumulating evidence that drug injectors will modify their behavior to reduce their risks for contracting AIDS. The earliest studies conducted in New York City reported that many sought sterile injection equipment, reduced the number of individuals with whom they shared needles, and reduced or ceased drug injection.[23] Similarly, two San Francisco community outreach projects reported that many injectors had adopted the use of bleach to sterilize their injection equipment.[24] Reductions in the AIDS-related sexual risk behaviors of injection drug users have been reported as well, albeit of lesser magnitude than reductions reported for drug-injection-associated risk behaviors.[25]

Based on these and other reports, in 1987 the National Institute on Drug Abuse initiated the multi-site National AIDS Demonstration Research (NADR) effort to develop and test the efficacy of various HIV risk-reduction intervention models. This was designed to provide rapid response to the critical need for detailed knowledge on how to achieve optimum effectiveness in reducing HIV-related risk behaviors among drug injectors utilizing minimal resources and brief interventions. The NADR projects were directed mainly at injection drug users who were not in drug treatment programs (estimated at the time to be approximately 85 percent of the total target population), as well as their sexual partners. By 1989, NADR projects were operational at 41 sites throughout the United States and Puerto Rico, and some of their many common features included the use of recovering addicts as outreach workers, HIV testing, a brief ("standard") or a more complex ("enhanced") risk reduction regimen, and follow-up.[26]

While all programs encouraged cessation of drug use, prudence dictated a working assumption that this would not be an immediate or uniform outcome. Therefore, the interventions also promoted such safer injection practices as eliminating needle sharing, using sterile injection equipment, and cleaning needles and syringes with bleach when sterile equipment was not available. With abstinence from sex as neither a realistic nor psycho-socially preferred goal, the projects universally encouraged safer sexual practices, such as reducing the number of sexual partners, avoiding drug-injecting partners, and using condoms during every sexual encounter. Many of the intervention project sites distributed condoms and/or bleach to study participants.

The Miami NADR project implemented one of the more comprehensive models, and its effectiveness has been well documented.[27] It focused on neighborhoods where the prevalence of drug abuse was particularly high. In addition, the research team collaborated with ethnographers who had extensive experience and contacts in the Miami drug scene and who were able to provide firsthand accounts of drug-taking activities in local shooting galleries and crack houses. These data emphasized the importance of hiring outreach workers similar in gender and ethnicity to the targeted subgroups and indigenous to the neighborhoods selected as recruitment sites. Ethnographic information also suggested the advisability of providing specialized interventions to specific subgroups, such as female sexual partners, Hispanics, and participants whose HIV tests were positive.

A risk-reduction pamphlet promoting needle cleaning and safer sexual behavior was produced in a colorful comic book format for distribution to participants and potential participants in the study. It presented a soap opera vignette of a young inner-city woman taking greater control of her life, and was pretested in the target community and through focus groups for accuracy of street language and images prior to its dissemination.

Indigenous outreach workers approached potential participants in street settings to encourage them to enroll in the intervention program. At the project's assessment center, at a location convenient to the recruitment sites, those agreeing to participate in the project received a pre-test counseling session during which the HIV testing procedure and the possible test results were explained. Following the blood test, a detailed health survey was administered to assess AIDS-related drug and sexual risk behaviors. Study participants were then randomized into "standard" or "enhanced" intervention groups. Standard intervention participants returned two weeks after their initial assessment to receive post-test counseling and the results of their HIV test. Following Centers for Disease Control protocols and National Institute on Drug Abuse guidelines, post-test counseling included information on the meaning of the test results, the modes of HIV transmission, and a thorough discussion of risk-reduction strategies. A packet of brochures was also given to each standard intervention participant, containing information about AIDS, injection drug users' risks for AIDS, drug treatment, general health facts, and social and health services available in the community.

Participants in the enhanced intervention also received the pre- and post-test counseling and educational brochures plus an additional four hours of group counseling divided into three sessions. This enhanced intervention was designed to take participants through a sequence of acquiring knowledge about HIV transmission, developing practical risk reduction skills (needle cleaning and condom use), empowering attitudinal and behavioral change, and developing a realistic plan to accomplish and maintain these changes.

After 24 months of observation, both the standard and enhanced intervention groups exhibited substantial and sustained reductions in

AIDS-related risk behaviors. Although there were no practical differences in the behavioral changes of one group when compared to the other, risk reductions were particularly evident in the area of drug use. An obvious conclusion of the effort is that intervention programs targeting injection drug users and their sex partners must concentrate efforts within the neighborhoods where participants reside or frequent. Cultural knowledge and sensitivity to ethnic considerations are necessary elements of any risk-reduction program. The use of indigenous outreach workers from the same racial/ethnic background as the target population was undoubtedly a major factor in the success of this program.

Effective intervention programs must focus on both drug-using and sexual behaviors and provide motivating information. Also, they must guide the development of specific technical and interpersonal skills that can provide the tangible means for changing high-risk behaviors. These skills need to be demonstrated in role playing sessions that mimic real-life situations as much as possible. Such programs must also be concerned with maintaining behavioral change once such change has been achieved.

CONDOMS—MALE AND FEMALE

Most everyone has heard of condoms, also known as bags, baggies, scum bags, rubbers, and skins.* The condom is a thin latex or membranous sheath worn over the penis during intercourse as a contraceptive device and/or for the prevention of sexually transmitted diseases. In history and folklore, the term "condom" has been attributed to a certain "Dr. Condom," reputedly a physician in the court of King Charles II of England (1630–1685) who developed it to control the number of illegitimate offspring being sired by His Majesty.[28] Or alternatively, John S. Farmer and William E. Henley's *Slang and Its Analogues*, published in seven volumes between 1890 and 1904, refers to the "cundum" as an obsolete appliance so-called from the name of its inventor, a colonel in the Guards of Charles II.[29] Interestingly, there is no mentioning of either the condom or the cundum in the respected *Oxford Dictionary of English Etymology*,[30] but the term most likely comes from the Latin *condus*, a receptacle.

---

*Over the years, condoms have also been referred to as balloons, bishops, buckskins, cheaters, condos, condominiums, diving suits, dreadnoughts, eel skins, envelopes, fish skins, French letters, French safes, Frenchies, frogs, frog skins, Italian letters, jo-bags, johnnies, joy bags, letters, lubies, one-piece overcoats, phallic thimbles, Port Said garters, prophos, raincoats, safes, safeties, safety sheaths, shower caps, and spitfires. See Richard A. Spears, *Slang and Euphemism* (Middle Village, NY: Jonathan David Publishers, 1981), p. 121.

The Male Condom

The condom is not a new invention. It has been reported that the early Egyptians used animal membranes to cover the penis, and in 1504 the Italian anatomist Gabriel Fallopius designed a medicated linen sheath that was pulled on over the penis.[31] The first dictionary to discuss the condom was Captain Francis Grose's *A Classical Dictionary of the Vulgar Tongue*, published in London in 1785. Capt. Grose had the following entry:

> *Cundum*. The dried gut of a sheep, worn by men in the act of coition, to prevent venereal infection; said to have been invented by one Colonel Cundum. These machines were long prepared and sold by a matron of the name of Phillips at the Green Canister, in Half-moon St., in the Strand.[32]

The earliest rubber condom carried a seam along its entire length, and was likely uncomfortable for all parties involved. Hand-dipping with glass formers began during the latter part of the nineteenth century, and the continuous production process in which formers are dipped in latex and then cured dates from the 1930s. Electronic testing of condoms (for leakage and breakage) was introduced in 1951, silicon lubricants were offered in the 1960s, and spermicidally lubricated condoms became available in 1975.[33]

How popular condoms were in past years would be difficult to reckon. What is clear, however, is that prior to the age of AIDS, they were continuously maligned. In 1667, Rochester, Roscommon, and Dorset—three aristocratic British courtiers, wits, and poets—issued their *A Panegyroc Upon Cundum*, satirically eulogizing the penile device.[34] In his *Memoirs*, the eighteenth-century Italian adventurer and rogue Giovanni Casanova likened the condom to an English overcoat. Furthermore, it was only as recently as 1977 that the United States Supreme Court abolished state laws that restricted the advertisement and display of condoms.

Since the emergence of AIDS, condoms have come from behind the counter and are sold openly—even having entire retail shops devoted exclusively to their promotion and sale. For the wearer, condoms provide a mechanical barrier that greatly reduces the risk of infections acquired through penile exposure to infectious cervical, vaginal, vulvar, or rectal secretions or lesions. For the wearer's partner, the proper use of condoms prevents semen deposition, contact with urethral discharge, and exposure to lesions on the head or shaft of the penis. In study after study, condoms have been found to be effective in the prevention and transmission of HIV.[35]

The Female Condom

An estimated 3 million women worldwide have HIV infection, with AIDS having become the leading cause of death among women between the ages of 20 to 40 in major cities throughout sub-Saharan Africa, Western Europe, and the Americas.[36] In the United States, women still represented but a small percentage (11.2 percent) of the cumulative AIDS cases as of late 1993.[37] Moreover, of the approximately 47,000 Americans who were diagnosed with AIDS during 1992, the great majority were males. However, while AIDS is still concentrated among gay and bisexual men and injection drug users, the new prevalence data suggest the direction that the epidemic is headed. While men who have sex with men experienced a decline in new cases, women reflected a sizable increase, and for the first time ever, sex surpassed injection equipment sharing as women's leading risk factor for AIDS.

There are indications that many of the traditional HIV prevention/intervention programs have not had a major impact in reducing high-risk sexual behaviors among women. Data from several of the National Institute on Drug Abuse's National AIDS Demonstration Research (NADR) projects, for example, have documented that increased AIDS education is not sufficient to reduce HIV risk behaviors.[38] Moreover, increased knowledge about HIV transmission, AIDS, and associated risk behaviors does not appear to bring about major reductions in sexual risk behaviors among those women who are at the greatest risk for HIV acquisition and transmission. This finding is apparent among numerous groups of women at high risk for HIV infection, including prostitutes contacted on the street,[39] heroin-addicted prostitutes,[40] incarcerated women,[41] arrestees,[42] and women of color.[43]

One of the difficulties is that risk-reduction methods are often not feasible for women at greatest risk for HIV infection. To date, the most common and effective risk-reduction method is condom use. However, many women report not using condoms on a regular basis, particularly with regular sex partners.[44] The lack, or irregular use, of condoms is typically related to social and lifestyle circumstances. For example, condom use is more likely to occur with women who are confidant in their negotiating power during sexual encounters.[45] However, many women at risk are unable to negotiate or insist on condom use with their partners.[46] This inability to insist on condom use results partially from some women's dependence on sex for drugs or money. Customers and sex partners frequently refuse to use a condom.[47] Moreover, insistence on condom use may result in violence. In addition, the drug abuse and addiction common to many of these women result in sex without condoms with injection drug users.

The risk factors associated with HIV acquisition and transmission specific to women are multiple and interrelated. Sex without condoms represents a risk for acquiring HIV.[48] However, the higher levels of unsafe sex associated with drug use increase the potential for infection by sex-for-crack exchanges,[49] with injection drug users,[50] and with numerous anonymous partners.[51] In fact, studies indicate that drug use may overshadow sexual activity as a risk factor for HIV.[52]

In addition, women's health status is strongly associated with risk. Women with a sexually transmitted disease (STD) who have sex without a condom are more suspectable to HIV infection than women who do not have an STD.[53] Other research substantiates the STD/drug use connection. Women who use crack are more likely to have STDs than those who do not.[54] Crack-using women also have a greater likelihood of high-risk sexual behaviors; they are less likely to use condoms and more likely to have numerous sex partners.

Socioeconomic circumstances have also been associated with increased risk of HIV infection. Poor women are at greater risk than middle- or upper-class women.[55] Women who are dependent on trading sex to support themselves increase their risk of HIV acquisition.[56] For many women of color, particularly those of low socioeconomic status, AIDS is only one of many life problems and often is rated by them as being less serious an issue than unemployment, lack of access to child care, and crime victimization.[57] Therefore, prevention/intervention as well as methods of risk reduction must take into account the entire life circumstances of women if these means are to be successful.

To date, there are few prevention/education programs tailored specifically for women that address the entire life spectrum, and developing such programs is one of the greater challenges facing prevention experts since so many issues must be addressed. For instance, women need to be educated on how to use condoms with regular sex partners. This often means incorporating changes into long-standing practices. As noted earlier in this chapter, it may also introduce mistrust into a relationship. Similarly, women need to be taught how to negotiate safe sex, particularly in situations where insistence on condom use may result in physical abuse or even serious violence.[58] Education programs need to address sexually transmitted diseases, their diagnosis and treatment, and their relationship to HIV acquisition and transmission. Many women, particularly African Americans and Latinas, as well as HIV-positive women, are less likely to have access to health-care services. Therefore, education programs need to teach women how to take advantage of these services, including using limited resources to obtain appropriate care. Prevention/intervention programs must be culturally sensitive, and they must be administered by culturally competent health educators, who will take into consideration the traditional gen-

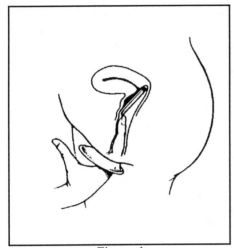

Figure 1
Female Condom Insertion

der roles as well as culturally specific gender roles of African-American and Latina women.

Perhaps most importantly, there are few women-controlled methods of sexual risk reduction available to women at risk of HIV infection, and what is available is not effective in preventing HIV infection. For example, both the effectiveness and the side effects of spermicides have raised questions about their feasibility as an HIV risk-reduction technique.[59] Sponges and diaphragms are promoted as HIV risk-reduction mechanisms because they reduce the incidence of STDs.[60] However, neither have actually been tested in terms of HIV-infection risk reduction. Yet, developing and promoting an effective woman-controlled risk-reduction method is essential if HIV acquisition and transmission are to be reduced among women at high risk.

Recently, such a method has become available—the Reality™ Vaginal Pouch, or simply, the female condom. The first female condom, made of rubber with a steel coil rim, was introduced in the 1920s.[61] However, it was not until the late 1980s that a more acceptable device was developed—the Femidom™ female condom, which has been commercially available in the United Kingdom since September 1992 and received FDA approval in the United States in 1993. In the United States, the female condom is marketed by Wisconsin Pharmacal Co. under the name of Reality™ effective mid-1994. The Reality™ female condom is a polyurethane sheath with a flexible inner ring that secures the condom against the cervix and an outer ring that prevents the condom from entering the vaginal canal. The design combines features of the male condom and the diaphragm.[62]

The female condom has several advantages over the male condom both as a contraceptive and as an STD-prevention method. First, it is woman-controlled. With the female condom, women are not as dependent on the cooperation of sex partners to protect themselves from HIV and other sexually transmitted diseases. Second, the female condom is inserted before intercourse, providing additional protection against infections from pre-ejaculated fluids. Third, the female condom protects a greater proportion of the vagina, providing additional protection against STDs. Fourth, the Reality™ condom has less risk of rupture than the male condom.[63] Other advantages are that, because of its loose fit, it causes less loss of sensitivity, it permits penetration before complete erection of the penis, and it permits continued intimacy in the resolution phase of intercourse since it need not be removed immediately.

Various tests have been performed on the Reality™ female condom with promising results. In a leak test where condoms were tested for pin holes and tears during manufacturing, Reality™ received a .6 percent leakage rate compared to a 3.5 percent leakage rate for the male condom. In another leak test measuring spillage during use, Reality™ had a 2.7 percent vaginal exposure rating whereas the male condom had a 8.1 percent rating. In 74 episodes in which Reality™ was used, there was no incidence of semen in the vagina. The combined risk for Reality™ is 3.0 percent and for the male condom 11.6 percent.[64] Furthermore, in other tests there was no viral leakage from Reality™.[65]

Several studies have tested the acceptability of Reality™ among both women and men. Of 24 couples studied in the United Kingdom, 67 percent of the women and 83 percent of the men found the female condom easy to use; 50 percent of the women and 54 percent of the men found it an acceptable contraceptive and HIV/STD prevention method; 50 percent of the women and 37 percent of the men preferred it to the male condom.[66] In a study of 294 American women, 73 percent found Reality™ easy to use; 56 percent considered it an acceptable contraceptive; and 82 percent found it an acceptable HIV/STD prevention method.[67] Another U.S. study examined the attitudes toward and acceptance of Reality™ among minority women. The sample included 20 African-American and 37 Latina women in a methadone maintenance program. The respondents did not use the condom but were interviewed on their acceptance of it after being educated about it. Over 75 percent of the women had favorable attitudes toward Reality™, 63 percent of their steady partners had favorable attitudes, and 65 percent of the women thought Reality™ would be easier to use than the male condom.[68]

To date, only two studies of the acceptability of the Reality™ female condom have been conducted among women at high risk for HIV, and in both instances the samples were extremely small. In Thailand, for example, 20 sex workers were educated about and given female condoms. The female condom was used in 32 percent of all sexual encounters and male condoms in 35 percent of sexual encounters. Almost all the women—90 percent—said they would recommend the female condom to friends.[69] Elsewhere, 24 prostitutes in Mexico were educated about the female condom. Twenty-one agreed to use it and 18 were interviewed at a later date about acceptance and use. After becoming accustomed to using the female condom, respondents felt it to be more protective against HIV and STD infection. The respondents also found female condoms more feasible to use than male condoms in that the former were more adaptable to their lifestyle. For example, respondents successfully learned to hide the outer ring of the female condom from clients to avoid discussion of condom use.* Many of the respondents used the female condom with regular sex partners, and both the respondents and their regular partners found the female condom acceptable.[70]

Previous research suggests promising results and high acceptability among diverse female populations with varying sexual histories and current practices. However, these studies have been on a small scale and additional data are needed to test the acceptability and efficacy of female condom use. Moreover, no studies have been conducted in the United States among women at high risk for HIV infection. These women would include prostitutes, injection drug users, or those who exchange sex for drugs. How the new female condom will fare among them, and in the general population as a whole, remains to be seen.

NEEDLE EXCHANGE

During the latter half of the 1980s, a number of AIDS prevention programs in the United States went beyond education and behavioral change strategies to include such proactive intervention techniques as distributing needle-cleaning supplies, latex condoms, and establishing needle exchange centers.

In Europe, many needle exchange programs were organized early in the AIDS epidemic. Several of them have been evaluated and were found to be somewhat effective.[71] The first needle exchange program began in the Netherlands in 1984. According to its founders, the rate of increase of infection among intravenous drug users slowed significantly after its inception.[72] Positive evaluations were also reported for a British program initiated two years after the Dutch piloted their experiment,[73] and other needle exchange programs have reported similar successes.[74]

In the United States, state and county government-approved needle exchange programs did not begin until 1988, the delay due mainly to the illegal status of needles and syringes in most parts of the country. In the overwhelming majority of state jurisdictions, injection equipment may not be legally purchased without a doctor's prescription. However, privately funded activist groups began distributing sterile

---

*This was accomplished by pushing the outer ring into the vagina and then pulling it back out immediately prior to intercourse.

equipment as early as 1986. Among the first was that operated by John Parker, a graduate student at Yale University. In 1986, Parker founded the Boston AIDS Brigade and began distributing needles in those neighborhoods with high rates of injection drug use.[75] He secured his needles legally in Vermont and transported them to Boston for distribution.

Since then, several legally sanctioned needle exchange programs have been implemented in the United States, beginning with a pilot program in New York City.[76] Other cities commenced similar operations, such as that developed in Tacoma, Washington. In January 1989, the Tacoma-Pierce health department added a needle exchange component to its drug education, counseling, and treatment programs.[77] Both the New York and Tacoma programs were designed to provide injection drug users with sterile needles in exchange for their used ones, and to monitor client samples to measure program effectiveness.

In general, studies of needle exchange programs indicate that 1) they are successful in reducing HIV risk behaviors; 2) there is no evidence that the programs increase injection drug use; 3) in some cases drug use actually declines; and, 4) they serve as valuable links to treatment, especially since many of the participants have never had contact with drug treatment programs.

The most publicized evaluation targeted New Haven's needle exchange program.[78] The program exchanged needles on a one for one basis with a maximum of five per visit. A first time client without a needle to exchange was given one "starter" needle. While the program was anonymous, all clients were given an ID number and a fake nickname. All needles dispensed were numbered, and these numbers were recorded in the client's file. Returned needles were counted and examined to see if the original client returned the needle. "Dedicated" clients were those who always returned the needles dispensed directly to them. A portion of the needles were also tested for the presence of HIV. The return rate was about 52 percent, and needles used by those considered "dedicated" clients had the lowest prevalence of HIV. They found that 91.7 percent of shooting gallery needles, 67.5 percent of street needles, and 50.3 percent of study needles tested positive for HIV antibodies. Moreover, the study reported that some 35 percent of dispensed needles were shared (i.e., not returned by the same person to which the needle was originally dispensed), a rate not much lower than the 39 percent who reported sharing needles during the seven-month period prior to the program sign-up. Finally, a fourth of those in the needle exchange program sought drug-abuse treatment, and of these, 57 percent were admitted to programs.

From the outset, however, needle exchange programs have been mired in controversy.[79] Some observers feared a repeat performance of the black-market diversion incidents that plagued methadone maintenance programs.[80] In April 1989, New York Congressman Charles Rangel introduced a bill banning federal funds or assistance to exchange programs and others that dispensed sterilizing materials. Rangel argued that:

> [A]ddicts . . . think that their habit is safe [when the government provides the needles] . . . this lends an air of approval to a practice that prolongs drug addiction.[81]

Also, there were claims that distribution of sterile needles enabled addicts to keep their habits, which—given their higher rates of injection drug use—amounted to genocide of African Americans and Hispanics.[82] In response to these accusations, exchange advocates pointed to statistics from the apparently successful projects elsewhere in the world that suggested that since the exchanges began, treatment entries increased and the rate of AIDS infection stabilized.[83]

The effectiveness of some needle exchange programs was called into serious question, however, often as an outgrowth of program policies. New York City's exchange program required that clients participating in the project carry identification cards, be in drug treatment, and travel significant distances to the program center. Participants received only one free needle at each visit to the center. This eliminated injection drug users with no money for transportation or no desire to enter treatment. Or as one intravenous drug user in New York remarked in late 1988:

> Who the hell are they trying to attract? There are what you could call your "good junkies," and there are your average, run-of-the-mill New York dope fiends. The good junkies who might be interested in the [needle] exchange already clean their needles, or don't mix blood in them, or don't share, and stuff like that. But then there are your street dope fiends, which are probably 99 percent of New York's junk heads. They want to be out in the street shooting and hustling, and that's why they're not in treatment. And besides, they wouldn't even cross the street to get a clean needle, no less cross town to get one. And then if from some miracle they did, they'd probably use it 'till it got dull, and then wrap it up in cellophane and sell it as new.[84]

Most critical of the needle exchange programs was the Bush administration,[85] but such official criticism began to change with the election of Bill Clinton in 1992. Clinton's first "AIDS czar," Christine Gebbie, was a strong supporter of needle exchange.[86] Furthermore, a University of California study sponsored by the Centers for Disease Control and Prevention called for a repeal of the ban on the use of federal funds for needle exchange services.[87] The report contained some important conclusions as well:

- By September 1, 1993, at least 37 active needle exchange programs existed in the United States.

- About one-half of the needle exchange programs in the United States are legal, but funding is often unstable and most programs rely on volunteer services to operate. All but six U.S. needle exchange programs rely on volunteer services to operate, all but six require one-for-one exchanges, and rules governing the exchange of syringes are generally well enforced.

- In addition to having distributed over 5.4 million syringes, U.S. needle exchange programs provide a variety of services ranging from condom and bleach distribution to drug treatment referrals.

- Some needle exchange programs have made significant numbers of referrals to drug abuse treatment and other public health services, but referrals are limited by the paucity of drug-treatment slots. Integrating needle exchange programs into the existing public health system is a likely future direction for these programs.

- Although needle-exchange program clients vary from location to location, the programs generally reach a group of injection drug users with long histories of injecting and who remain at significant risk for HIV infection. Needle exchange program clients, furthermore, have had less exposure to drug-abuse treatment than those not using the programs.

- The majority of studies of needle exchange program clients demonstrate decreased rates of HIV drug-related risk behaviors, but not decreased rates of sexual risk behaviors.

- Studies of the effect of needle exchange programs on injection-related infectious diseases other than HIV provide limited evidence that the programs are associated with reductions in subcutaneous abscesses and hepatitis B among injection drug users.

- Multiple mathematical models addressing the potential impact of needle exchange programs suggest that programs can prevent significant numbers of infections among their clients, as well as clients' drug and sex partners, and their children. In almost all cases, the cost per HIV infection averted is far below the $119,000 lifetime cost of treating an HIV-infected person.

As an outgrowth of the apparent success of needle exchange programs, in mid-1994 the National Academy of Sciences panel discussed earlier in this chapter strongly recommended lifting the ban on the use of federal funds for needle exchange programs.[88]

POSTSCRIPT

The impact of a decade of AIDS prevention/intervention efforts has been decidedly mixed. Many injection drug users have refrained from using shooting galleries, no longer share needles, and/or have adopted safer needle use practices. However, many continue to share other types of injection paraphernalia, such as cookers, cottons, and rinse water, which are often contaminated, or they share potentially HIV-contaminated drugs through backloading and frontloading practices.[89] Among those who have made significant progress in reducing their drug use-related HIV risk behaviors, many continue to engage in a variety of risky sexual practices.

Perhaps the most notable gains in reducing sexual risks have occurred among gay and bisexual men, with significant proportions reducing their numbers of sexual partners, maintaining monogamous relationships, and/or using condoms on a regular basis. Yet a disturbing trend in the gay community has been increasing rates of unprotected anogenital intercourse among younger men, and relapse to unsafe sex among older men.[90] Many gay men, saying that they are numb with loss, fatalistic about their own survival, unwilling to face a measure of sexual deprivation, and aware of the attention showered on the sick and the dying, are again practicing unprotected anal intercourse. A gay man recently encountered in a Miami sex club explained:

> No matter what, we're all going to get it [AIDS]. With my identity as gay and AIDS so entwined, believe it or not I'm kind of attracted to the idea of testing positive and getting sick. All the guilt associated with my friends dying will go away, and I'll have a better sense of belonging. Maybe the KS [Kaposi's sarcoma] will be a badge of honor that will give my life some meaning.

In the general population, much progress needs to be made. A recent survey found that between 15 and 31 percent of heterosexuals nationally, and between 20 and 41 percent in cities with a high incidence of AIDS, reported at least one HIV risk factor. Condom use was relatively low—practiced *all of the time* by only 17 percent of those with multiple sex partners, 13 percent of those with risky sexual partners, and 11 percent of transfusion recipients who had not been tested for HIV.[91]

Quite clearly, there are major segments of the population that have not been reached by prevention programs. Among these are heterosexual, non-drug-using adolescents and college students who do not perceive themselves to be at risk. In addition, it would appear that the development of techniques for both motivating and sustaining behavioral changes should be a major priority.

END NOTES

1. John Ciardi, *A Browser's Dictionary: A Compendium of Curious Expressions and Intriguing Facts* (New York: Harper & Row, 1980), p. 253.

2. Gina Kolata, "Prospects for AIDS Vaccine Dim as New Tests Show Wide Failures," *The New York Times*, 13 November 1993, p. 11.

3. Peter H. Duesberg, "HIV Is Not the Cause of AIDS," *Science*, 241 (1988), pp. 514–516.

4. See Gary P. Wormser (ed.), *AIDS and Other Manifestations of HIV Infection* (New York: Raven Press, 1992).

5. *U.S. News & World Report*, 9 August 1993, p. 55.

6. Martin Fishbein, "Testimony Before the National Commission on AIDS," Austin, Texas, 10 March 1993.

7. *Behavioral and Social Sciences and the HIV/AIDS Epidemic* (Washington, DC: National Commission on AIDS, 1993), p. 3.

8. Committee on Substance Abuse and Mental Health Issues in AIDS Research, Institute of Medicine, National Academy of Sciences, *AIDS and Behavior: An Integrated Approach* Washington, DC: National Academy Press, 1994).

9. "Understanding AIDS: An Informational Brochure Being Mailed to All U.S. Households," *Morbidity and Mortality Weekly Report*, 37 (6 May 1988), pp. 261–262.

10. For example, see John V. Flowers, Curtis Booraem, Timothy E. Miller, Annette E. Iverson, John Copeland, and Ken Furtado, "Comparison of the Results of a Standardized AIDS Prevention Program in Three Geographic Locations," *AIDS Education and Prevention*, 3 (1991), pp. 189-196; M. Campbell and W. Waters, "Public Knowledge About AIDS Increasing," *British Medical Journal*, 294 (1987), pp. 892–893; Marshall H. Becker and Jill G. Joseph, "AIDS and Behavioral Change to Reduce Risk: A Review," *American Journal of Public Health*, 78 (1988), pp. 394-410.

11. M.C. Donoghoe, G.V. Stimson, and K.A. Dolan, "Sexual Behavior of Injecting Drug Users and Associated Risks of HIV Infection for Non-injecting Sexual Partners," *AIDS Care*, 1 (1989), pp. 51-58.

12. Ron D. Stall, Thomas J. Coates, and Colleen Hoff, "Behavioral Risk Reduction for HIV Infection Among Gay and Bisexual Men," *American Psychologist*, 43 (1988), pp. 878–885.

13. John B. Jemmott, Loretta S. Jemmott, and Geoffrey T. Fong, "Reductions in HIV Risk-Associated Sexual Behaviors Among Black Male Adolescents: Effects of an AIDS Prevention Intervention," *American Journal of Public Health*, 82 (1992), pp. 372-377.

14. Jeffrey A. Kelly, Janet S. St. Lawrence, Harold V. Hood, and Ted L. Brasfield, "Behavioral Intervention to Reduce AIDS Risk Activities," *Journal of Consulting and Clinical Psychology*, 57 (1989), pp. 60-67.

15. Flowers et al.

16. Jeffrey A. Kelly and Janet S. St. Lawrence, "The Impact of Community-Based Groups to Help Persons Reduce HIV Infection Risk Behaviours," *AIDS Care*, 2 (1990), pp. 25–35.

17. Suzanne E. Landis, JoAnne L. Earp, and Gary G. Koch, *AIDS Education and Prevention*, 4 (1992), pp. 61–70.

18. G. S. Martin, G. Serpelloni, U. Galvan, A. Rizzetto, M. Gomma, S. Morgante, and G. Rezza, "Behavioural Change in Injecting Drug Users: Evaluation in an HIV/AIDS Education Programme," *AIDS Care*, 2 (1990), pp. 275–279.

19. Nancy S. Padian, Thomas R. O'Brien, YoChi Chang, Sarah Glass, and Donald P. Francis, "Prevention of Heterosexual Transmission of Human Immunodeficiency Virus Through Coups Counseling," *Journal of Acquired Immune Deficiency Syndromes*, 6 (1993), pp. 1043–1048.

20. J. A. Wiley and M. C. Samuel, "Prevalence of HIV Infection in the USA," *AIDS*, 3 (1989), Supplement 3, pp. S71–S78.

21. M. Marmor, K. Krasinsky, M. Sanchez, H. Cohen, N. Dubin, L. Weiss, A. Manning, N. Saphier, C. Harrison, and D. J. Ribble, "Sex, Drugs, and HIV Infection in a New York City Hospital Population," *Journal of Acquired Immune Deficiency Syndromes*, 3 (1990), pp. 307–318.

22. R. Conviser and J. H. Rutledge, "The Need for Innovation to Halt AIDS Among Intravenous Drug Users and Their Sexual Partners," IV International Conference on AIDS, Stockholm, 12-16 June 1988.

23. Don C. Des Jarlais, Samuel R. Friedman, and William Hopkins, "Risk Reduction for the Acquired Immunodeficiency Syndrome Among Intravenous Drug Users," *Annals of Internal Medicine*, 313 (1985), pp. 755–759; Samuel R. Friedman, Don C. Des Jarlais, and J. Sotheran, "AIDS Health Education for Intravenous Drug Users," *Health Education Quarterly*, 13 (1986), pp. 383–393; P. A. Selwyn, C. Feiner, C. P. Cox, C. Lipshutz, and R. L. Cohen, "Knowledge About AIDS and High-Risk Behavior Among Intravenous Drug Users in New York City," *AIDS*, 1 (1987), pp. 247–254.

24. John K. Watters, "A Street-Based Outreach Model of AIDS Prevention for Intravenous Drug Users: Preliminary Evaluation," *Contemporary Drug Problems*, 14 (1987), pp. 411–423; A. R. Moss and R. E. Chaisson, "AIDS and Intravenous Drug Use in San Francisco," *AIDS and Public Policy Journal*, 3 (1988), pp. 37–41.

25. See Charles F. Turner, Heather G. Miller, and Lincoln E. Moses (eds.), *AIDS: Sexual Behavior and Intravenous Drug Use* (Washington, DC: National Academy Press, 1989).

26. For a detailed examination of the entire NADR effort, see Barry S. Brown and George M. Beschner (eds.), *Handbook on Risk of AIDS: Injection Drug Users and Sexual Partners* (Westport, CT: Greenwood Press, 1993).

27. Clyde B. McCoy, James E. Rivers, and Elizabeth L. Khoury, "An Emerging Public Health Model for Reducing AIDS-Related Risk Behavior Among Injecting Drug Users and Their Sexual Partners," *Drugs and Society*, 7 (1993), pp. 143–159; Dale D. Chitwood, James A. Inciardi, Duane C. McBride, Clyde B. McCoy, H. Virginia McCoy, and Edward Trapido, *A Community Approach to AIDS Intervention: Exploring the Miami Outreach Project for Injecting Drug Users and Other High Risk Groups* (Westport, CT: Greenwood Press, 1991).

28. Hugh R. K. Barber, "Condoms (Not Diamonds) Are a Girl's Best Friend," *Female Patient*, 15 (1990), pp. 14–16.

29. John S. Farmer and W. E. Henley, *Slang and Its Analogues, Past and Present: A Dictionary, Historical and Comparative, of the Heterodox Speech of*

All Classes of Society for More Than Three Hundred Years, Vol. II (New York: Arno Press, 1970, reprint of the 1891 edition), p. 229.

30. C. T. Onions (ed.), *The Oxford Dictionary of English Etymology* (New York: Oxford University Press, 1966).

31. Barber.

32. Francis Grose, *A Classical Dictionary of the Vulgar Tongue* (London: C. Chappel, 1785).

33. Malcolm Potts and Roger V. Short, "Condoms for the Prevention of HIV Transmission: Cultural Dimensions," *AIDS,* 3 (1989, Supp. 1), pp. S259–S263.

34. See Eric Partridge, *The Macmillan Dictionary of Historical Slang* (New York: Macmillan, 1973), p. 231.

35. For example, see Roger Detels, Patricia English, Barbara R. Visscher, Lisa Jacobson, Lawrence A. Kingsley, Joan S. Chmiel, Janice P. Dudley, Lois J. Eldred, and Harold M. Ginzburg, "Seroconversion, Sexual Activity, and Condom Use Among 2,915 HIV Seronegative Men Followed for Up to Two Years," *Journal of Acquired Immune Deficiency Syndromes,* 2 (1989), pp. 77–83; Joseph A. Catania, Thomas J. Coates, Susan Kegeles, Mindy Thompson Fullilove, John Peterson, Barbara Marin, David Siegel, and Stephen Hulley, "Condom Use in Multi-Ethnic Neighborhoods of San Francisco: The Population-Based AMEN (AIDS in Multi-Ethnic Neighborhoods) Study," *American Journal of Public Health,* 82 (1992), pp. 284–286; John L. Peterson, Thomas J. Coates, Joseph A. Catania, Lee Middleton, Bobby Hilliard, and Norman Hearst, "High-Risk Sexual Behavior and Condom Use Among Gay and Bisexual African-American Men," *American Journal of Public Health,* 82 (1992), pp. 1490–1494; J. B. F. de Witt, T. G. M. Sandford, E. M. M. de Vroome, G. J. P. van Griensven, and G. J. Kok, "The Effectiveness of Condom Use Among Homosexual Men," *AIDS,* 7 (1993), pp. 751–752.

36. James Chin, "Current and Future Dimensions of the HIV/AIDS Pandemic in Women and Children," *The Lancet,* 336 (1990), pp. 221–227; Catherine A. Hankins and Margaret A. Handley, "HIV Disease and AIDS in Women: Current Knowledge and a Research Agenda," *Journal of Acquired Immune Deficiency Syndromes* 5 (1992), pp. 957–971.

37. Centers for Disease Control and Prevention, *HIV/AIDS Surveillance Report,* 5 (October 1993), p. 6.

38. James L. Sorensen, Laurie A. Wermuth, David R. Gibson, Kyung-Hee Choi, Joseph R. Guydish, and Steven L. Batki, *Preventing AIDS in Drug Users and Their Sexual Partners* (New York: Guilford Press, 1991); Gloria Weissman, and the National AIDS Research Consortium, "AIDS Prevention for Women at Risk: Experience from a National Demonstration Research Program," *Journal of Primary Prevention,* 12 (1991), pp. 49–63; Chitwood et al.

39. Nzilambi Nzila, Marie Laa, Manoka Abib Thiam, Kivuvu Mayimona, B. Edidi, Eddy Van Dyck, Frieda Behets, Susan Hassig, Ann Nelson, K. Mokwa, Rhoda L. Ashley, Peter Piot, and Robert W. Ryder, "HIV and Other Sexually Transmitted Diseases Among Female Prostitutes in Kinshasa," *AIDS* 5 (1991), pp. 715–721.

40. David J. Bellis, "Fear of AIDS and Risk Reduction Among Heroin-Addicted Female Street Prostitutes: Personal Interviews with 72 Southern California Subjects," *Journal of Alcohol and Drug Education*, 35 (1990), pp. 26–37.

41. Jennifer Davis-Berman and Debra Brown, "AIDS Knowledge and Risky Behavior by Incarcerated Females: IV and Non-IV Drug Users," *Social Science Review*, 75 (1990), pp. 8–11.

42. Joseph B. Kuhns and Kathleen M. Heide, "AIDS-Related Issues Among Female Prostitutes and Female Arrestees," *International Journal of Offender Therapy and Comparative Criminology*, 36 (1992), pp. 231–245.

43. Adeline Nyamathi, Crystal Bennett, Barbara Leake, Charles Lewis, and Jacquelyn Flaskerud, "AIDS-Related Knowledge, Perceptions, and Behaviors among Impoverished Minority Women," *American Journal of Public Health*, 83 (1993), pp. 65–71.

44. Nancy S. Padian, "Prostitute Women and AIDS: Epidemiology." *AIDS*, 2 (1988), pp. 413–419; Robert F. Schilling, Nabila El-Bassel, Louisa Gilbert, and Steven P. Schinke, "Correlates of Drug Use, Sexual Behavior, and Attitudes Toward Safer Sex Among African-American and Hispanic Women in Methadone Maintenance," *Journal of Drug Issues*, 21 (1991), pp. 685–698; Ronald O. Valdiserri, Vincent C. Arena, Donna Proctor, and Frank A. Bonati, "The Relationship Between Women's Attitudes About Condoms and Their Use: Implications for Condom Promotion Programs," *American Journal of Public Health*, 79 (1989), pp. 499–501.

45. William P. Sacco, Brian Levine, David L. Reed, and Karla Thompson, "Attitudes About Condom Use as an AIDS-Relevant Behavior: Their Factor Structure and Relation to Condom Use," *Psychological Assessment: A Journal of Consulting and Clinical Psychology*, 3 (1991), pp. 265–272.

46. Dooley Worth, "Sexual Decision-Making and AIDS: Why Condom Promotion Among Vulnerable Women is Likely to Fail," *Studies in Family Planning*, 20 (1989), pp. 297–307; Michael J. Rosenberg, Arthur J. Davidson, Jian-Hua Chen, Franklyn N. Judson, and John M. Douglas, "Barrier Contraceptives and Sexually Transmitted Diseases in Women: A Comparison of Female-Dependent Methods and Condoms," *American Journal of Public Health*, 82 (1992), pp. 669–674; Stephanie Kane, "AIDS, Addiction and Condom Use: Sources of Sexual Risk for Heterosexual Women," *Journal of Sex Research*, 27 (1990), pp. 427–444.

47. James A. Inciardi, Dorothy Lockwood, and Anne E. Pottieger, *Women and Crack-Cocaine* (New York: Macmillan, 1993).

48. Michael J. Rosenberg and Jodie M. Weiner, "Prostitutes and AIDS: A Health Department Priority?" *American Journal of Public Health*, 78 (1988), pp. 418–423.

49. H. Virginia McCoy and James A. Inciardi, "Women and AIDS: Social Determinants of Sex-Related Activities," *Women and Health*, 20 (1993), pp. 69–86; Carole A. Campbell, "Prostitution, AIDS, and Preventive Health Behavior," *Social Science Medicine*, 32 (1991), pp. 1367–1378; Marsha F. Goldsmith, "Sex Tied to Drugs = STD Spread," *Medical News and Perspectives*, 260 (1988), p. 2009.

50. Nancy J. Padian, J. Carlson, R. Browning, L. Nelson, J. Grimes, and L. Marquiss, "Human Immunodeficiency Virus (HIV) Among Prostitutes in Nevada," *Third International Conference on AIDS*, Washington, D.C., June 1987.

51. Harvey A. Siegal, Robert G. Carlson, Russel Falick, Mary Ann Forney, Jichuan Wang, and Ling Li, "High-Risk Behaviors for Transmission of Syphilis and Human Immunodeficiency Virus Among Crack Cocaine-Using Women," *Sexually Transmitted Diseases,* 19 (1992), pp. 266–271; Moira L. Plant, Martin A. Plant, David F. Peck, and Jo Setters; "The Sex Industry, Alcohol and Illicit Drugs: Implications for the Spread of HIV Infection," *British Journal of Addiction,* 84 (1989), pp. 53–59; Inciardi, Lockwood, and Pottieger.

52. Robert E. Fullilove, Mindy Thompson Fullilove, Benjamin P. Bowser, and Shirley A. Gross, "Risk of Sexually Transmitted Disease Among Black Adolescent Crack Users in Oakland and San Francisco," *Journal of the American Medical Association,* 263 (1990), pp. 851–855; Robert T. Rolfs, Martin Goldberg, and Robert G. Sharrar, "Risk Factors for Syphilis: Cocaine Use and Prostitution," *American Journal of Public Health,* 80 (1990), pp. 853–857.

53. Padian 1988.

54. Sevgi O. Aral and King K. Holmes, "Sexually Transmitted Diseases in the AIDS Era," *Scientific American,* 264 (1991), pp. 62–69.

55. Vivian T. Shayne and Barbara J. Kaplan, "Double Victims: Poor Women and AIDS," *Women and Health,* 17 (1991), pp. 21–37.

56. Worth 1989; Campbell 1991.

57. Seth C. Kalichman, Tricia L. Hunter, and Jeffrey A. Kelly, "Perceptions of AIDS Susceptibility Among Minority and Nonminority Women at Risk for HIV Infection," *Journal of Consulting and Clinical Psychology,* 60 (1992), pp. 725–732.

58. Zena A. Stein, "HIV Prevention: The Need for Methods Women Can Use," *American Journal of Public Health,* 80 (1990), pp. 460–462.

59. Zena A. Stein, "Editorial: The Double Bind in Science Policy and the Protection of Women from HIV Infection," *American Journal of Public Health,* 82 (1992), pp. 1471–1472.

60. Michael J. Rosenberg and Erica L. Gollub, "Commentary: Methods Women Can Use That May Prevent Sexually Transmitted Disease, Including HIV," *American Journal of Public Health,* 82 (1992), pp. 1473–1478.

61. Editorial, "The Female Condom," *British Journal of Family Planning,* 18 (1992), pp. 71–72.

62. Walli Bounds, "Male and Female Condoms," *British Journal of Family Planning,* 15 (1989), pp. 14–17.

63. Mary Ann Leeper and M. Conrardy, "Preliminary Evaluation of REALITY: A Condom for Women to Wear," *Advances in Contraception,* 5 (1989), pp. 229–235; Walli Bounds, John Guillebaud, Laura Stewart, and Stuart Steele, "A Female Condom (Femshield): A Study of Its User Acceptability," *British Journal of Family Planning,* 14 (1988), pp. 83–87; Erica L. Gollub and Zena A. Stein, "Commentary: The New Female Condom—Item I on a Women's AIDS Prevention Agenda," *American Journal of Public Health,* 83 (1993), pp. 498–500.

64. Mary Ann Leeper, "Preliminary Evaluation of REALITY, A Condom for Women to Wear," *AIDS Care,* 2 (1990), pp. 287–290.

65. Bruce Voeller, "Gas, Dye, and Viral Transport Through Polyurethane Condoms," *Journal of the American Medical Association,* 266 (9119), pp. 2986–

2987; W. Lawrence Drew, Margaret Blair, Richard C. Miner, and Marcus Conant, "Evaluation of the Virus Permeability of a New Condom for Women," Unpublished Manuscript from the Mount Zion Hospital and Medical Center, Biskind Pathology Research Laboratory, San Francisco, California; and the University of California, San Francisco, California.

66. Robert F. Schilling, Nabila El-Bassel, Mary Ann Leeper, and Linda Freeman, "Acceptance of the Female Condom by Latin- and African-American Women," *American Journal of Public Health*, 81 (1991), pp. 1345–1346.

67. Schilling et al. 1991.

68. Schilling et al. 1991.

69. C. Sakondhavat, "Further Testing of Female Condoms," *British Journal of Family Planning*, 15 (1990), p. 129.

70. Mauricio Hernandez-Avila, "Report to Wisconsin Pharmacal Company: Acceptability of Female Condoms Among Female Prostitutes in Mexico City—Preliminary Findings." Communication to Dr. Mary Ann Leeper from Dr. Mauricio Hernandez-Avila, Director, Center for Public Health Research, National Institute of Public Health, Mexico, 17 March 1992.

71. C.A. Raymond, "U.S. Cities Struggle to Implement Needle Exchanges Despite Apparent Successes in European Cities," *Journal of the American Medical Association*, 260 (1988), pp. 2620–2621.

72. E. Buning, T. Reid, H. Hagan, and L. Pappas, "Needle Exchange V: Update on the Netherlands and the United States," *Newsletter of the International Working Group on AIDS and IV Drug Use*, 4 (June 1989), pp. 9–10; C. Hartgers, E. C. Buning, G. W. Van Santen, A. D. Verster, and R. A. Coutinho, "The Impact of the Needle and Syringe-Exchange Programme in Amsterdam on Injecting Risk Behavior," *AIDS* 3 (1989), pp. 571–576.

73. *The New York Times*, 29 Feb. 1988, p. A4; *Alcoholism and Drug Abuse Week*, 26 April 1989, p. 5.

74. G. V. Stimson, "Editorial Review: Syringe-Exchange Programmes for Injecting Drug Users," *AIDS*, 3 (1989), pp. 253–260; M. C. Donoghoe, G. V. Stimson, K. Dolan, and L. Alldritt, "Changes in HIV Risk Behavior in Clients of Syringe-Exchange Schemes in England and Scotland," *AIDS*, 3 (1989), pp. 267–272; G. J. Hart, A. L. M. Carvell, N. Woodward, A. M. Johnson, P. Williams, and J. V. Parry, "Evaluation of Needle Exchange in Central London: Behaviour Change and Anti-HIV Status Over One Year," *AIDS*, 3 (1989), pp. 261–265; *World Press Review*, June 1988, pp. 31–32.

75. *International Journal On Drug Policy*, September/October 1989, p. 5.

76. C. A. Raymond, "First Needle Exchange Program Approved: Other Cities Await Results," *Journal of the American Medical Association*, 259 (1988), pp. 1289–1290.

77. *Alcoholism and Drug Abuse Week*, 12 July 1989, p. 7; *The New York Times*, 23 Jan. 1989, p. A12.

78. Elaine O'Keefe, Edward Kaplan, and Kaveh Khoshnood, *City of New Haven Needle Exchange Program: Preliminary Report* (New Haven, CT: City of New Haven's Mayor's Office, 1991).

79. See, "Needle Exchange Goes on Trial," *International Journal On Drug Policy*, 1 (1989), p. 5.

80. B.T. Farid, "AIDS and Drug Addiction Needle Exchange Schemes: A Step in the Dark," *Journal of the Royal Society of Medicine*, 81 (1988), pp. 375–376.

81. *Alcoholism and Drug Abuse Week*, 26 April 1989, p. 5.

82. *Drug Abuse Report*, 22 Nov. 1988, p. 1.

83. Hartgers et al.

84. For a full commentary and chronology of the New York program, see *The New York Times*, 1 Jan. 1988, p. A1; *Time*, 15 Feb. 1988, p. 81; *The New York Times*, 6 June 1988, p. B3; *The New York Times*, 8 Nov. 1988, pp. B1, B5; *The New York Times*, 13 Nov. 1988, p. E6; *The New York Times*, 30 Jan. 1989, p. A1; C. Gilman, "After One Year: New York City's Needle Exchange Pilot Programme." *International Journal On Drug Policy* 1 (1990), pp. 18–21.

85. Office of National Drug Control Policy, *Needle Exchange Programs: Are They Effective?* (Washington DC: Executive Office of the President, 1992).

86. *Newsweek*, 9 August 1993, p. 62.

87. *The Public Health Impact of Needle Exchange Programs in the United States and Abroad* (Berkeley and San Francisco: University of California, 1993).

88. Committee on Substance Abuse and Mental Health Issues in AIDS Research.

89. Benny Jose, Samuel R. Friedman, Alan Neaigus, Richard Curtis, Jean-Paul C. Grund, Marjorie F. Goldstein, Thomas P. Ward, and Don C. Des Jarlais, "Syringe-Mediated Drug Sharing (Backloading): A New Risk Factor for HIV Among Injection Drug Users," *AIDS*, 7 (1993), pp. 1653–1660.

90. Robert B. Hays, Susan M. Kegeles, and Thomas J. Coates, "High HIV Risk-Taking Among Young Gay Men," *AIDS*, 4 (1990), pp. 901–907; Susan Kippax, June Crawford, Mark Davis, Pam Rodden, and Gary Dowsett, "Sustaining Safe Sex: A Longitudinal Study of a Sample of Homosexual Men," *AIDS*, 7 (1993), pp. 279–282; John B.F. de Witt, Johanna A. R. van den Hoek, Theo G. M. Sandfort, and Godfried J. P. van Griensven, "Increase in Unprotected Anogenital Intercourse Among Homosexual Men," *American Journal of Public Health*, 83 (1993), pp. 1451–1453; John B. F. de Witt, Godfried J. P. van Griensven, Gerjo Kok, and Theo G. M. Sandfort, "Why Do Homosexual Men Relapse Into Unsafe Sex? Predictors of Resumption of Unprotected Anogenital Intercourse With Casual Partners," *AIDS*, 7 (1993), pp. 1113–1118.

91. Thomas J. Coates, "Prevention of HIV-1 Infection: Accomplishments and Priorities," *Journal of NIH Research*, 5 (July 1993), pp. 73–76.

Viral Evolution and *Behavioral* Quarantine

In 1954 Jack Finney wrote a science-fiction novel titled *The Body Snatchers*. The first film version of the story came two years later as *The Invasion of the Body Snatchers*, starring Kevin McCarthy. There was a remake in 1978 with Donald Sutherland and Brooke Adams; and just as everyone thought it was safe to take a nap, a third version was released in 1994 (as *Body Snatchers*) with Meg Tilly and Gabrielle Anwar (Al Pacino's dance partner in *Scent of a Woman*). It was the story of alien seed "pods" which exuded blank human forms that drained the emotional life of people, taking over their bodies, and in so doing destroying both personality and individuality. Most interesting was how those who were still "normal" would peer intently at one another as if to detect the telltale change, the sign that one had "crossed over" and had become one of "them"—alien and lethal. *The Body Snatchers* offered a vivid example of the plague mentality.

In the plague mentality, one belongs to the kingdom of life or the kingdom of death. The mentality developed during the great bubonic plague of the fourteenth century.[1] People were afraid to approach one another, parents abandoned children, wives left husbands, and all normal social relationships stopped. It is said, too, that when children in the streets saw the telltale signs of the plague, they sang "Ring around a rosie!" The lyric meant that they saw a ring on the skin that surrounded a red spot—an indication of the onset of the disease. "A pocket full of posies" stood for the fresh flowers that plague victims carried to mask the stench of the disease. Then there was the apocalyptic ending to the verse: "All fall down." The Black Death ultimately took one-fifth of the population of Western Europe.[2]

Despite its rather benign-sounding acronym, AIDS has rekindled aspects of the plague mentality. The recognition of AIDS as a new disease phenomenon was initially quite confusing and perplexing. To

149

those physicians who first observed an extraordinarily rare form of skin malignancy—Kaposi's sarcoma—occurring in a cluster of young gay men, it appeared that a "gay cancer" had surfaced in the United States. To those who began reporting unprecedented concentrations of a peculiar form of pneumonia—also within the gay community—it seemed that they were encountering what the media later called a "gay plague." However, when reports began surfacing of cases with similar manifestations occurring in groups as diverse as intravenous drug users of both sexes, heterosexual Haitian immigrants, hemophiliac recipients of blood-clotting material, infants of affected mothers, and odd cases that failed to fit into any of the other groups, it quickly became clear that AIDS was anything but a homosexual epidemic.

Although there have been far more pervasive epidemics, the initial association of AIDS with homosexuals created a population of "new untouchables." As reports of AIDS spread and it became apparent that other populations were involved as well, irrational fear, paranoia, and discrimination tended to abound. Haitians and homosexuals have suffered employment and housing discrimination as a result of their association with the disease. Many children infected with HIV, even those who have not become AIDS symptomatic, are shunned from classrooms, play groups, and foster homes. Prisoners with AIDS are being segregated from other inmates, and in some jurisdictions, local jails have their "leper cells" in which AIDS cases are segregated. Throughout the world, Africans, Haitians, Americans, and all others associated with the virus have become the targets of a new type of xenophobia.

The manner in which the plague mentality will continue to flow through and expand in populations untouched by HIV and AIDS is difficult to predict. The method is dependent on the future course of the epidemic, the progress of HIV vaccine research, the effectiveness of prevention and control efforts, and the politics of AIDS in government and the media.

THE ACCELERATION OF AIDS

One of the first recorded outbreaks of a new epidemic disease occurred in Athens, Greece, in 430 B.C. Aspects of the affliction were described by Thucydides in his celebrated *History of the Peloponnesian War*:

> First, overwhelming fever in the head and redness . . . of the eyes came over them; the throat and tongue became blood red. From these beginnings there ensued sneezing and hoarseness, and in short order the distress settled in the chest with a violent cough, and there followed the emesis of every kind of bile. The skin was flushed, livid, and broken with

small blisters and open sores. The patient burned with fever, and most perished of the fever in the ninth or the seventh day.

Although there is disagreement as to the cause of the Athenian plague,[3] it is speculated that it was a form of influenza complicated by staphylococcal toxic shock syndrome. Importantly, it was a new disease, and it had a mortality rate of 33 percent.

The bubonic plague of the Middle Ages, also known as the "Black Death," the "Great Dying," and the "Great Pestilence," lasted from 1346 to 1352. Most scholars agree that it initially erupted on the Asian steppes as an epidemic among marmots. Trappers collected the fur of the dead animals and sold them in bales to buyers from the West, and, presumably, ravenous fleas jumped from the bales to human hosts.[4] Having a mortality rate of between 70 percent and 80 percent, during the six years that the plague endured it killed some 20 million people.

Still vivid in the minds of a few Americans is the epidemic of "Spanish Flu" that occurred in 1918–1919. Although influenza is now considered a somewhat benign affliction, the strain that emerged early in this century was particularly virulent, killing between 20 and 40 million people worldwide.[5] In the United States, 25 million people caught the disease, and 500,000 perished from it. As a young physician in Fort Devens, Massachusetts first described it:

> These men start with what appears to be an ordinary attack of influenza, and when brought to the hospital they very rapidly develop the most vicious type of pneumonia. Two hours after admission they have the mahogany spots over the cheek bones, and a few hours later you can begin to see the cyanosis [bluish skin discoloration] spreading all over the face. It is only a matter of hours until death comes, and it is simply a struggle for air until they suffocate.[6]

The Athenian plague of the fifth century B.C. and the bubonic plague of the Middle Ages moved with a comparative slowness. They inched across the land and sea with plodding caravans and sailing ships or at the pace of such other carriers as rats and insects. The Black Death, for example, took 14 years to move from East Asia to England. The early-twentieth-century influenza epidemic, with more modern forms of transportation available, moved quite rapidly. The epidemic is believed to have begun in March of 1918 when a U.S. Army cook at Fort Riley, Kansas, complained of chills and fever—the familiar symptoms of flu.[7] By the end of the week, 522 others were reporting similar symptoms, and 46 eventually died. But the deaths were attributed to complications brought about by pneumonia, not flu. Moreover, with the United States fully immersed in World War I, Camp Riley continued to train and ship army recruits across the Atlantic. When they arrived in France, the flu accompanied them—a lethal stowaway—and spread across Europe, and then to Russia, India, China, Japan, Africa,

South America, and even to Alaska and Samoa. While it was devastating, the epidemic was blessedly short. By the beginning of 1919, it was virtually gone.

In contrast with AIDS, however, most epidemic diseases have a short incubation period, and run their course fairly quickly. AIDS, on the other hand, has a long incubation period. After transmission and initial infection with HIV, the disease produces no distinctive symptoms, sometimes for 10 or more years. But in the meantime, those infected can transmit the virus to others, an so on in turn. The average time between the onset of symptoms and the total collapse of the immune system is three to four years. And death is a virtual certainty. AIDS, indeed, is a slow but steady plague, and with 40 million infections expected by the year 2000, it will be the most pervasive and costly epidemic in history.

One of the factors that will contribute to the acceleration of AIDS is the action of other sexually transmitted diseases in potential hosts. That a history of sexually transmitted disease increases the likelihood of infection when exposed to HIV has been known for some time. In 1993, however, it became clearer that syphilis, gonorrhea, chancroid, and other STDs can increase the risk of HIV infection as much as a hundredfold. Studies conducted at the Institute of Tropical Medicine in Antwerp, Belgium, suggested two mechanisms of this synergistic reaction.[8] The first is that the inflammation associated with the presence of STDs increases the production of infection-fighting white blood cells, which can break down the mucous membranes in the genitals. Because some varieties of these cells are also the key targets of HIV, their presence increases the pool of cells that are vulnerable to attack. Alternatively, genital infections increase white blood cells in semen and vaginal secretions. Thus, an HIV-positive sex partner infected with another STD carries more infected cells, and poses a greater risk of infection for the other partner.

For heterosexuals who view AIDS as a disease limited to gay and bisexual men, injection drug users, prostitutes, and inner-city and Third World populations, consider the following. In 1993, a study by the Alan Guttmacher Institute found that more than one in five of all Americans—some 56 million people—are infected with a viral sexually transmitted disease; that 12 million new sexually transmitted diseases occur each year in the United States (two-thirds of them to people under age 25 and one quarter to teenagers); and that sexually transmitted diseases affect women disproportionately, because women tend to show fewer infections and thus go untreated for longer periods.[9] *What these data suggest is that a higher proportion of American men and women are at a greater risk for HIV infection than they believe.*

VIRAL EVOLUTION AND
THE FUTURE OF HIV

New infectious diseases do not appear to evolve through the spontaneous generation of new microbes from some fundamental, primordial clutter. Rather, they generally arise by cross-species transmission of relatively benign, nonpathogenic agents from animal reservoirs. In the history of medical science there are many documented instances of humans becoming infected with a virus from an animal species, either directly by close contact or indirectly through an insect vector. This has been the case with the herpes viruses, such alpha viruses as Western and Venezuelan encephalitis, and the influenza viruses to name but a few.[10]

A recent example of an infectious disease emerging from an animal reservoir occurred during the late spring of 1993 in the Southwestern corner of the United States. Beginning in May of that year, cases of acute illness characterized by fever, headache, muscle pain, coughing, and lung congestion were reported by the Indian Medical Center in Gallup, New Mexico. After the initial flu-like symptoms, the malady would quickly worsen. Lung tissue would fill with fluid, and patients would literally drown in their own body fluids. More than half the cases were ending in death.[11] Health officials referred to it as UARDS, for Unexplained Adult Respiratory Distress Syndrome; others called it "Four Corners disease," because it was initially identified in the region around the intersection of Arizona, New Mexico, Colorado, and Utah. In time, the disease was named Hantavirus Pulmonary Syndrome (HPS), and its source was found to be the wild deer mouse.

It is unlikely that HPS was an entirely new syndrome. People die of respiratory infections all the time, and some cases are labeled as "unexplained." Moreover, hantavirus-related diseases have been reported since the 1930s, with manifestations similar to those observed in the Southwestern United States. The reason why the 1993 outbreak was severe enough to be noticed was relatively clear. Heavy rains produced an unusually rich crop of piñon nuts—a staple in the deer mouse nutritional fare. This, in turn, triggered an explosion in the mouse population. When the rodents urinate or defecate, the virus is spread into soil or dust that can be inhaled by humans. By the close of 1993, with the help of concerted public health education and rodent extermination campaigns, the prevalence of new cases of HPS had declined dramatically.[12]

Although the explicit origin of AIDS remains undetermined, it is now generally accepted that the current epidemic has its origins in African non-human primates.[13] These primates seem to act both as natural, asymptomatic (without symptoms) hosts of a wide family of immunodeficiency viruses ("simian immunodeficiency viruses" or SIV) and as potential reservoirs for further transmission to humans. Analyses of stored blood samples drawn from patients throughout North America, Europe, and Africa early in this century seem to indicate that an SIV-like virus began infecting humans between 50 and 100 years ago.[14] In 1984, the first simian immunodeficiency virus was isolated, and it was found to be widespread among African green monkeys in the wild. Currently, on the basis of seroepidemiological data, it appears that there may be as many as 30 distinct types of SIV harbored in their African monkey hosts. Interestingly, when comparing the SIV encountered in West African sooty mangabey monkeys with HIV-2, the variety of human immunodeficiency virus found in West Africa, the two cannot be immediately differentiated.[15] Only through patient analyses of their genetic material does it become evident that they are not quite the same.

As for the cross-species leap, there is only speculation—interspecies sex, vaccine contamination, or perhaps rituals involving injections of monkey blood (inadvertently contaminated with SIV) into humans to heighten sexual arousal.[16] The truth, however, as suggested earlier in this book, is likely far more mundane. Many African tribes hunt monkeys and butcher them for meat; others keep them as pets. In either case, it is easy to imagine being cut by a hunting knife or being bitten by a pet; such incidents are followed by the introduction of monkey blood or other fluids through the wound opening.

While the origins of AIDS remain cloudy, the future of the virus is even less clear. What is known, however, is that viruses mutate constantly, evolving tens of thousands times faster than plants or animals, and that HIV mutates faster than most other viruses. In fact, HIV's mutation speed may be the reason why neither a cure nor an effective vaccine have been found. When confronted by a new drug or immune reaction, the virus quickly mutates out of its range.

Perhaps HIV is not a new and inherently deadly virus, after all, but an old one that has recently acquired deadly tendencies. Charles Darwin demonstrated how species evolve through natural selection, changing their character to adapt to their environments. When they do not adapt, they become extinct. HIV's success has been its mutability, as a result of outside pressures.

A variation of this perspective has been offered by Amherst College biology professor Paul Ewald.[17] Ewald's thesis is based on several assumptions:

- HIV existed in a benign state for decades, perhaps even centuries, before it started causing AIDS;

- it remained benign because it was sequestered in remote communities, confined to isolated groups having no carriers to other populations;

- replication and mutation into an aggressive form was unlikely under these circumstances, because doing so would have decimated HIV's host population, and itself in the process;

- when social changes occurred that provided HIV with access to other populations, more virulent and deadly forms of the virus evolved.

Within this context, and assuming that the current AIDS epidemic originated in Africa, as most epidemiologists agree, there were indeed social changes in many African nations that hastened the spread of HIV. As discussed briefly in Chapter One, starting in the 1960s such things as war, tourism, and commercial trucking forced the outside world on Africa's once isolated villages. At the same time, drought and industrialization prompted mass migrations from the countryside to the growing cities. Also, as the French medical historian Mirko Grmek has noted, urbanization shattered the social structures that constrained sexual behavior.[18] Prostitution increased and venereal diseases flourished, and at about the same time the use of hypodermic needles and mass inoculations became widespread. Taking this perspective even further, the global economy and air transport systems combined to hasten the diffusion of HIV and AIDS to other parts of the world, increasing the number of communities through which the virus could easily spread. The sexual revolution of the 1960s had broken down many of the barriers to monogamy in segments of the heterosexual population, and the gay liberation movement of the 1970s had a major impact on sexual practices in male homosexual communities. Finally, laws controlling the availability of hypodermic needles in the United States and the existence of shooting galleries and needle sharing provided HIV with easy access to injection drug users as viral hosts.

If this thesis is of any merit, and the deadliness of HIV is a result of its rapid spread, it would seem logical that with the right pressures the virus might grow less pernicious, that with a slowing of the spread of HIV it might evolve into a more benign form. In the absence of a cure or a palliative vaccine, there are only two mechanisms. The first is *prevention* through abstinence, condom use, or monogamy with regard to sexual behavior; and drug treatment, needle exchange programs, and the proper cleaning of drug paraphernalia among injection drug users. The other is *"behavioral* quarantine," a sequestering of the behaviors that contribute to the spread of HIV. Even if the thesis of viral evolution is without merit, the same alternatives remain—prevention and *behavioral* quarantine.

BEHAVIORAL QUARANTINE

Lew Wallace's *Ben-Hur: A Tale of Christ*[19] is the story of Judah Ben-Hur, a Jewish patrician youth who is falsely accused by his former friend Messala of attempting to murder the Roman governor of Judea. He is sent to the galleys for life, and his mother and sister are imprisoned. Escaping, Ben-Hur returns as a Roman officer and enters the chariot race in which Messala has wagered heavily on himself. Messala hopes to ruin Ben-Hur, but instead is seriously injured. His cruelties are discovered, and he is slain by his wife, Isas. Ben-Hur rescues his mother and sister, now lepers, and all are converted to Christianity after the disease is cured through the intervention of Jesus.

In the 1959 MGM motion-picture version of *Ben-Hur*, a frightening portrait of leprosy was presented to international audiences. For eight years Ben-Hur's mother and sister had been imprisoned in a leper's cell, where they caught the dreaded disease. Upon their release they were forced to leave Jerusalem and take refuge in the "city of lepers," a dwelling place for the "accursed of God." As presented in *Ben-Hur*:

> Possibly the reader does not know all the word [lepers] means. Let him be told it with reference to the Law of the time.
>
> "These four are accounted dead—the blind, the leper, the poor, and the childless." Thus the Talmud.
>
> That is, to be a leper was to be treated as dead—to be excluded from the city as a corpse; to be spoken to by the best beloved and most loving only at a distance; to dwell with none but lepers; to be utterly underprivileged; to be denied the rites of the Temple and the synagogue; to go about in rent garments and with covered mouth, except when crying, "unclean, unclean!" to find home in the wilderness or in abandoned tombs; to become a materialized specter of Himmon and Gehenna; to be at all times less a living offence to others than a breathing torment to self; afraid to die, yet without hope except in death.[20]

AIDS is viewed by many as the late-twentieth-century version of leprosy,* and has led to many discussions about quarantining those

---

*Leprosy is a chronic, mildly infectious and communicable disease caused by the microorganism, *Mycobacterium leprae*. The disease is marked by nodules on the surface of the body which, if left untreated, can ultimately cause ulcerations, deformities, mutilations, and blindness. It is thought to be communicated chiefly by close contact for months or years with those already having the disease. However, specific methods of transmission and the degree of communicability and risk are poorly defined. The incubation period can range up to 20 years. Leprosy is also an ancient disease, and is believed to have existed in Egypt as early as 4000 B.C. The *Mycobacterium leprae* organism was identified in 1868 by the Norwegian physician Gerhard Hansen, which led to the adoption of "Hansen's disease" as a preferred designation for leprosy. Although it is treatable, it still occurs in tropical and subtropical communities where crowded and unsanitary conditions contribute to its spread, with Africa having two-thirds of all registered cases worldwide. In the United States Hansen's disease is found occasionally in California, Texas, Hawaii, Florida, and Louisiana, and infectious patients are cared for at the National infected with HIV.* Quarantine is perhaps the oldest form of public health regulation, with its roots dating back to the Old Testament.** The word comes from the Italian *quarantenaria* or the Latin *quadraginia*, meaning 40 days and referring to the 40-day detention placed on ships from plague-ridden ports during the late Middle Ages and Early Renaissance.[21] The term also refers to the isolation of individuals thought to have been exposed to contagious disease. Quarantine has been permissible by law in the United States for almost two centuries. In 1796, for example, the first federal quarantine law was passed in response to an epidemic of yellow fever.[22] In subsequent years, quarantine regulations were enacted and enforced typically under state and local law, and were considered both constitutional and advantageous to public health for the control such diseases as tuberculosis, small pox, and syphilis. For the better part of the twentieth century, however, given the great strides in medical science and therapy, quarantine laws have been little used, and the practice is generally considered to be archaic, excessive, and unnecessarily coercive.

Almost immediately after the discovery of AIDS, discussions of quarantine once more were being heard. Perhaps the most visible of those promoting quarantine was North Carolina Republican Senator Jesse Helms, who commented in 1987:

> I may be the most radical person you've talked to about AIDS, but I think that somewhere along the line we are going to have to quarantine, if we are really going to contain this disease.[23]

An AIDS quarantine could take several forms. A jurisdiction could (theoretically, at least) impose a quarantine on anyone who tested positive for HIV. Alternatively, the quarantine could focus only on those clinically diagnosed with AIDS. Finally, a jurisdiction could target only those with HIV or AIDS who refuse to stop engaging in activities that spread the disease. Any form of quarantine, however, poses a variety of problems.

Going beyond the civil rights and libertarian issues,*** isolating everyone testing positive for HIV would be costly, if possible at all.

Leprosarium in Carville, Louisiana. See Douglas B. Young and Stewart T. Cole, "Leprosy, Tuberculosis, and the New Genetics," *Journal of Bacteriology*, 175 (1993), pp. 1-6; S.G. Browne, "How Old Is Leprosy?" *International Journal of Dermatology*, 19 (1980), pp. 530-532; "WHO Vows to Eradicate Leprosy by Year 2000," *UN Chronicle*, September 1991, p. 64.

*For a comparison of AIDS and leprosy, see Ilse J. Volinn, "Issues of Definitions and Their Implications: AIDS and Leprosy," *Social Science and Medicine*, 29 (1989), pp. 1157-1162.

**For example, as stated in *Leviticus 13:46*: "He shall remain unclean all the days during which he has the infection; he is unclean. He shall live alone; his dwelling shall be outside the camp."

***For a thorough discussion of the civil liberties issues associated with quarantining those with HIV and AIDS, see Wendy E. Parmet, "AIDS and Quarantine: The Revival of

Those in the United States who are HIV positive number in the millions. How would they be identified, housed, cared for? The whole idea is so impractical, unrealistic, and preposterous that it warrants no further discussion. A quarantine targeting those with clinical AIDS would certainly be more pragmatic from a logistical point of view, but it would accomplish little. Such individuals represent but a small percentage of those capable of spreading the disease. Moreover, since they are "ill," they tend to be less likely to engage in risky behaviors than those without symptoms of the disease. Restraining HIV-infected prostitutes, injection drug users, and others who continue to engage in "risky" behaviors would accomplish little from a preventive point of view, since such "recalcitrant" individuals are comparatively few in number.

Rather than a *physical* quarantine of people, it can be argued that a *behavioral* quarantine of the virus might be more appropriate and manageable. Behavioral quarantining involves approaches which separate, segregate, and sequester behaviors that transmit HIV. Needle exchange programs represent a form of behavioral quarantine; so do the prohibitions against anal and oral sex in many contemporary gay bath houses and sex clubs. The "no condom, no sex" aphorism adopted by many prostitutes and others who have multiple sex partners is another type of behavioral quarantine. Perhaps the most inclusive form of behavioral quarantine exists in the blood-bank industry. At the Blood Bank of Delaware, for example, which is typical of others in the United States, the following "sensitive" questions are asked of every donor:

Have You Ever:

- Been diagnosed as having AIDS?
- Had sex with anyone who has had a positive test for the AIDS virus?
- Taken illegal drugs with a needle, even one time?
- Had sex with anyone who has ever taken illegal drugs with a needle?
- Taken clotting factor concentrates for a bleeding disorder such as hemophilia?
- Had sex with anyone who has taken clotting factor concentrates for a bleeding disorder such as hemophilia?
- Taken money or drugs for sex at any time since 1977?
- Given money or drugs to anyone to have sex with you at any time in the last 12 months?
- Had sex with a man who had sex, even one time since 1977, with another man? (Not applicable for males.)

an Archaic Doctrine," *Hofstra Law Review*, 14 (1985), pp. 53-90.

- Had sex with another man even one time since 1977? (Not applicable for females.)

An affirmative answer to even one of these questions disqualifies a person as a blood donor.

POSTSCRIPT

During the late spring and early summer of 1981, when researchers in Los Angeles and New York City were first reporting a new and distinct clinical entity associated with immune dysfunction among young gay men,[24] HIV infection and AIDS were already on an upward climb. Although the number of cases was small, evidence suggests that hundreds of thousands of infections had already occurred in North America, many urban areas of sub-Saharan Africa, and some parts of the Caribbean. HIV had also been introduced into the large cities in Western Europe and Oceania. But HIV and AIDS were not at all understood, and even if an HIV test had been available at the time, the testing of sexually active adults on a comprehensive scale would not have been possible. Moreover, restricting the travel and sexual practices of those identified as infected would have been equally infeasible. Thus, the national and global spread of HIV and AIDS could not have been prevented. However, it could have been dramatically slowed!

The mistakes made were many, including official indifference in many governmental quarters and many unfortunate political decisions—based more on ideology and fear than on humanitarian concerns and the best interests of public health. A key difficulty was associated with "Reaganism," "Reaganomics," the "New Federalism," and the whole Reagan agenda. Reaganism stressed economic individualism and a policy of cutting programs and taxes, increasing defense spending, reducing government regulation, and encouraging private investment by the wealthy so that the benefits would "trickle down" through the economy. Reaganism, furthermore, was not just the politics of President Reagan, but the whole ideological syndrome he epitomized. And there were other aspects to Reaganism. As author Dennis Altman commented:

> In the search to recreate the rest of the world in America's image and the domestic world in terms of traditional moral values, Reaganism seeks to escape the admittedly unpleasant realities of the present and to replace them with a mythical utopia of an America unchallenged in the world and held together by a common set of values at home.[25]

In retrospect, there was likely no one better qualified to lead America's charge back to the 1950s than the aging movie actor himself.

With regard to AIDS, Reaganism displayed rather obvious overtones of political discrimination. AIDS was perceived as a disease of gays and drug users—heavily tainted populations in the eyes of the Reagan White House, populations that might just disappear if they were ignored long enough. A uniquely unreserved glimpse into the Reagan administration's attitude toward the AIDS epidemic came on April 15, 1985, when U.S. Secretary of Health and Human Services Margaret Heckler commented, "We must conquer AIDS before it affects the heterosexual population."[26] Reagan's position on the matter was that "The Scriptures are on our side."[27]

In 1987, in what was described as just the first stage of the Reagan administration's *new* strategy to combat the AIDS epidemic, Attorney General Edwin Meese announced that all federal prisoners would henceforth be tested for HIV, and that the results of those tests might influence whether some prisoners would ever be granted parole. Meese explained:

> One of the factors on when people leave prison certainly has to do with whether they are a danger to the community.[28]

In the same speech, Meese also unveiled the new plan under which HIV-positive tourists, immigrants, and refugees would be denied entry into the United States.

Interestingly, in Ronald Reagan's 748-page autobiography, *An American Life*,[29] most of which is devoted to his eight years as President of the United States, the subject of AIDS is not mentioned even once. In Nancy Reagan's book, *My Turn*,[30] a 348-page memoir of her eight-year reign as First Lady, the word "AIDS" is mentioned only once. In connection with a brief discussion of Rock Hudson, she reflected:

> He had been to a White House dinner and had been at my table. I remember sitting across from him and thinking, Gee, he's thin. I asked if he had been dieting.

Mrs. Reagan gave far more attention to how desperately shabby the china and table cloths were in the White House when she first moved in than to the epidemic of our time.

The recalcitrance of the Reagan administration's position on AIDS, and that of George Bush's administration as well, was related not only to ideology but also to the fact that talking about AIDS meant talking about sex and drugs. Reagan and Bush found these areas to be awkward subjects, so they steered clear of them. This deliberate avoidance clearly served to fuel the epidemic. A clear policy combined with funding for research surely would have slowed the spread of HIV and AIDS. Moreover, the unwillingness of the Republican White House policymakers to support needle exchange programs hastened the spread of the epidemic among injection drug users and their sexual partners. And when billions of dollars were finally allocated for AIDS research, the overwhelming majority was put into the pursuit of an AIDS vaccine, a search for a "magic bullet." Comparatively minimal funding was targeted for education and prevention programs, and for social and behavioral research, which, in the long run, would have been far more cost-effective.

Given the past, where do we go from here? Several considerations seem warranted:

1. Since it is human behaviors that are driving the AIDS epidemic, funding for AIDS-related social science, behavioral, and prevention research should equal that of biomedical research.

2. The federal government and the great majority of state jurisdictions effectively encourage drug injectors to share needles, syringes, and other parts of the injection kit by treating the paraphernalia as contraband. Such laws should be altered, and needle exchange programs should be implemented wherever they are needed.

3. The Centers for Disease Control and Prevention (CDC) needs to be more explicit about sex in its AIDS prevention messages. The U.S. Congress, however, our sacred repository of culture lag, prohibits the CDC from using such words as "anal" and "vaginal." Such a suffocating posture has no place in the face of epidemic disease.

4. For injection drug users, and crack users who exchange sex for drugs, drug abuse treatment is likely the most effective mechanism of AIDS prevention. Thus, funding for drug abuse treatment, and treatment research, needs to be greatly increased.

5. For students, prisoners, and persons who cannot afford to purchase them, condoms should be made readily available on a widespread basis.

6. Since only men, women, and children can contract AIDS, no one is immune; as such, prevention messages must be continuous, targeting all population groups.

In the final analysis, one can only hope that AIDS will go the way of smallpox. The pockmarked, mummified face of Ramses V is mute testimony to the presence of the disease as far back as ancient Egypt. Once a vaccine was made widely available in the nineteenth century, smallpox was squeezed relentlessly into a smaller and smaller area by a successful worldwide vaccination campaign. In 1977 the last carrier was vaccinated, and smallpox was declared extinct by the World Health Organization in 1980. We can only hope that AIDS will not endure for as long as smallpox before it is finally conquered.

END NOTES

1. See Neil M. Ampel, "Plagues—What's Past is Present: Thoughts on the Origin and History of New Infectious Diseases," *Reviews of Infectious Diseases*, 13 (1991), pp. 658–665.

2. See William H. McNeill, *Plagues and Peoples* (Garden City, NY: Doubleday, 1976).

3. See A. D. Langmuir, T. D. Worthen, J. Solomon, C. G. Ray, and E. Petersen, "The Thucydides Syndrome: A New Hypothesis for the Cause of the Plague of Athens," *New England Journal of Medicine*, 313 (1985), pp. 1027–1030; A. J. Holladay, "The Thucydides Syndrome: Another View," *New England Journal of Medicine*, 315 (1986), pp. 1179–1173.

4. Ampel, p. 659.

5. Brian R. Murphy and Robert G. Webster, "Influenza Viruses," in Bernard N. Fields (ed.), *Virology* (New York: Raven Press, 1985), pp. 1179–1239.

6. Ampel, p. 659.

7. Peter Radetsky, *The Invisible Invaders: The Story of the Emerging Age of Viruses* (Boston: Little, Brown, 1991), p. 229.

8. Marie Laga, "STD Control for HIV Prevention," IX International Conference on AIDS, Berlin, 6-11 June 1993.

9. Felicity Barringer, "1 in 5 in U.S. Have Sexually Caused viral disease," *The New York Times*, 1 April 1993, p. A1.

10. Jonathan S. Allan, "Viral Evolution and AIDS," *Journal of NIH Research*, 4 (1992), pp. 51–54.

11. Centers for Disease Control and Prevention, "Outbreak of Acute Illness— Southwestern United States, 1993," *Morbidity and Mortality Weekly Report*, 43 (1993), pp. 421–424.

12. *Time*, 9 December 1993, p. 66.

13. Gerald Myers, Kersti MacInnes, and Bette Korber, "The Emergence of Simian/Human Immunodeficiency Viruses," *AIDS Research and Human Retroviruses*, 8 (1992), pp. 373–386.

14. Robin Marantz Henig, *A Dancing Matrix: Voyages Along the Viral Frontier* (New York: Alfred A. Knopf, 1993), p. 41.

15. Peter Gould, *The Slow Plague: A Geography of the AIDS Pandemic* (Oxford: Blackwell, 1993), p. 15.

16. Henig, p. 46.

17. Paul W. Ewald, "The Evolution of Virulence," *Scientific American*, April 1993, pp. 86–93.

18. Mirko D. Grmek, *History of AIDS: Emergence and Origin of a Modern Pandemic* (Princeton, NJ: Princeton University Press, 1990).

19. Lew Wallace, *Ben-Hur: A Tale of Christ* (New York: Harper & Brothers, 1900).

20. Wallace, Vol.II, pp. 626–627.

21. William H. McNeill, *Plagues and Peoples* (Garden City, NY: Doubleday, 1976).

22. *Act of May 27, 1796, Ch. 31, 1 Stat. 474*, cited in Wendy E. Parmet, "AIDS and Quarantine: The Revival of An Archaic Doctrine," *Hofstra Law Review*, 14 (1985), pp. 53–90.

23. *The New York Times*, 15 June 1987, p. 3.

24. Centers for Disease Control "Pneumocystis Pneumonia in Los Angeles," *Morbidity and Mortality Weekly Report*, 30 (5 June 1981), pp. 250–252; Centers for Disease Control, "Kaposi's Sarcoma and Pneumocystis Pneumonia Among Homosexual Men—New York City and California," *Morbidity and Mortality Weekly Report*, 30 (3 July 1981), pp. 305–308; M. S. Gottlieb, R. Schroff, H. Schanker, J. D. Weismal, P. T. Fan, R. A. Wolf, and A. Saxon, "Pneumocystis Carinii Pneumonia and Mucosal Candidiasis in Previously Healthy Homosexual Men: Evidence of a New Acquired Cellular Immunodeficiency," *New England Journal of Medicine*, 305 (10 Dec. 1981), pp. 1425–1431; H. Masur, M. A. Michelis, J. B. Greene, I. Onorato, R. A. Vande Stouwe, R. T. Holzman, G. Wormser, L. Brettmen, M. Lange, H. W. Murray, and S. Cunningham-Rundles, "An Outbreak of Community Acquired Pneumocystis Carinii Pneumonia: Initial Manifestation of Cellular Immune Dysfunction," *New England Journal of Medicine*, 305 (1981), pp. 1431–1438.

25. Dennis Altman, *AIDS in the Mind of America: The Social, Political, and Psychological Impact of a New Epidemic* (Garden City, NY: Doubleday/Anchor, 1987), p. 27.

26. Leigh W. Rutledge, *The Gay Decades: From Stonewall to the Present* (New York: Penguin Books, 1992), p. 239.

27. Rutledge, p. 250.

28. Rutledge, p. 275.

29. Ronald Reagan, *An American Life* (New York: Simon and Schuster, 1990).

30. Nancy Reagan, *My Turn: Memoirs of Nancy Reagan* (New York: Random House, 1989).

Name Index

Abdul-Quader, A., 118
Aboulafia, D., 60
Abrams, Donald L., 63
Adler, M.W., 115, 116
Adriaans, N.F.P., 64
Agar, Michael, 89
Alam, M., 60
Alesander, S.S., 26
Alexander, P., 117
Alizon, Marc, 27
Allan, Jonathon S., 162
Alldritt, L., 147
Allen, J.R., 115
Alroy, J., 27
Altman, Dennis, 25, 26, 28, 88, 163
Ampel, Neil M., 162
Anderson, R.E., 61
Andreani, T., 25
Antonelli, L., 119
Apertrei, Roxana C., 61
Aral, Sevgi, O., 146
Arena, Vincent C., 145
Armstrong, Donald, 25, 115, 119
Asbury, Herbert, 88
Asher, D.M., 27
Ashley, Rhoda L., 121, 144
Ashman, Margarita A., 80n., 89
Aubertin, P., 116
Auerbach, D.M., 25, 61

Baden, Michael M., 63
Bakalar, James B., 91, 118
Ball, John C., 118
Barber, Hugh R.K., 143, 144
Barnett, Tony, 116, 117, 121
Barre-Sinoussi, F.T., 63
Barringer, Felicity, 162
Bartlett, John G., 61
Basch, Paul F., 121
Bashur, R.I., 116
Bateson, Mary Catherine, 60
Batki, Steven L., 144
Batties, Robert J., 117
Bauer, Gary, 68

Bayer, Ronald, 88
Bazell, Robert, 21
Bebenroth, Donna, 119
Beck, E.J., 116
Becker, Marshall H., 142
Behets, Frieda, 121, 144
Beldescu, Nicolae, 61
Bellis, David J. 145
Bennett, Crystal, 145
Bennett, J.E., 24
Berkelman, Ruth L., 56, 57, 64
Berquist, R., 62
Beschner, George, 89
Bigelow, George E., 89
Biggar, R.J., 116
Billy, John O.G., 119
Bittencourt, Achilea L., 24
Black, David, 31n.
Blaikie, P., 116, 117, 121
Blair, Margaret, 147
Blanken, P., 64
Bodner, Anne J., 64
Bohmer, T. 26
Boite, C., 60
Bolan, Robert, 7
Bonati, Frank A., 145
Bonecker, C., 60
Bonneux, L., 115, 116
Booraem, Curtis, 142
Booth, R., 64
Bothwell, T.H., 27
Bottone, Edward J., 25, 64
Bounds, Walli, 146
Bourgois, Phillipe, 90
Bovelle, Elliott, 89
Bowmer, Ian, 121
Bowser, Benjamin P., 91, 118, 146
Brady, Elizabeth, 64
Braff, Irwin, 62
Brasfield, Ted L., 142
Brennan, R.O., 6n.
Brettle, R., 115, 116
Brettmen, L., 24, 163
Brinkley, David, 21-22

Brookmeyer, Ron, 61
Brooner, Robert K., 89
Brown, Barry S., 90, 143
Brown, Debra, 145
Brown, Lucille, 65
Browning, Frank, 62
Browning, R., 145
Brunham, R.C., 117
Bryant, Anita, 7-8
Buchbinder, S.P., 119
Bulkin, Wilma, 65
Buning, E.C., 147
Burke, D.S., 117
Bush, George, 23, 68, 160
Bush, Timothy J., 122
Butzler, Jean-Paul, 119
Byington, R., 115

Calabrese, L.H., 116
Calisher, Charles, 122
Calomfirescu, Alexandru, 61
Cameron, D.W., 116, 117
Campbell, M., 142, 145
Camus, Albert, vi-vii, viii
Cannon, L., 119
Cantwell, Alan, 17-18, 27
Capitani, C., 60
Cardon, B., 119
Careal, Michel, 119
Carlson, J., 145
Carlson, Robert G., 146
Carmen, A., 117
Carroll, Peter N., 25, 65
Carswell, J.S., 116, 117
Carvell, A.L.M., 147
Cassel, G.A., 27
Castro, Kenneth G., 122
Catania, Joseph A., 144
Ceausescu, Nicolae, 36, 37
Chaisson, R.E., 143
Chakrabarti, Lisa, 27
Chambers, Carl D., 118
Chang, YoChi, 143
Chardon, Claude, 12
Cheang, M., 117
Checquer, P., 120
Chen, Jian-Hua, 145
Chermann, J.C., 63
Cheynier, Remi, 27
Chiasson, Mary Ann, 90, 118
Chin, James, 60, 144

Chitwood, Dale D., 63, 80n., 89, 90, 118, 122, 143
Chmiel, Joan S., 144
Choi, Kyung-Hee, 144
Chu, Susan Y., 56, 57, 64
Ciardi, John, 123, 142
Clausen, L., 27
Clinton, Bill, 139
Clumeck, N.J., 26, 116, 119
Coates, Thomas J., 142, 144, 148
Cohen, C.S., 116
Cohen, H., 143
Cohen, J.B., 115, 117
Cohen, Jon, 28
Cohen, R.L., 143
Cohen, P.T., 117
Cole, Stewart T., 157n.
Cole, W.R., 26
Comerford, Mary, 80n., 89, 91, 122
Conant, Marcus A., 24, 147
Connally, John, 16n.-17n.
Conrardy, M., 146
Conviser, R., 143
Cookson, J., 27
Cooper, D.A., 63
Copeland, John, 142
Cornet, P., 115
Cortes, E., 60
Coulaud, J.P., 119
Coutinho, R.A., 119, 147
Cox, C.P., 143
Cran, S., 116
Crane, Lansing E., 89
Craven, D.E., 115
Crawford, D., 115
Crawford, June, 148
Crumley, Bruce, 120
Cunningham, D.G., 116
Cunningham-Rundles, S., 24, 163
Curran, J.W., 25, 61, 115
Curran, William J., 89
Curtis, Richard, 148
Curtis, Tom, 19-20, 27

Daniel, H., 121
Daniel, Muthiah D., 27
Darrow, W.W., 25, 61
Darwin, Charles, 154
Da Silva, Antusa A., 24
Davidson, Arthur J., 145
Davidson, S.J., 115, 116

Davis, Mark, 148
Davis-Berman, Jennifer, 145
D'Costa, Lourdes J., 117, 121
Delph, Edward W., 88
De Mol, Patrick, 116, 119
Des Jarlais, Don C., 65, 118, 143, 148
Desrosiers, Ronald C., 27
Detels, Roger, 60, 144
DeVita, Vincent T., 25, 26, 27, 61, 119
de Vroome, E.M.M., 144
de Witt, John B.F., 144, 148
Dickenson, G.M., 115
Dolan, K.A., 142, 147
Donegan, C., 116
Donoghoe, M.C., 142, 147
Doto, Irene, 62
Douglas, John M., 145
Douglous, G., 24
Dowsett, Gary, 148
Drake, W.L., 26
Drew, W. Lawrence, 147
Duberman, Martin, 61
Dubin, N., 143
Dudley, Janice P., 144
Duesberg, Peter H., 124, 142
Dugas, Gaetan, 11
Durack, D.T., 6n.
Duval, E., 119

Earp, JoAnne L., 143
Eckholm, Erik, 24, 60, 119
Edelman, Robert, 119
Edidi, B., 121, 144
El-Bassel, Nabila, 145, 147
Eldred, Lois J., 63, 144
El-Sadr, Waffa, 64
Elvin-Lewis, M., 26
Emeson, Eugene, 64
English, Patricia, 144
Essex, Max, 26
Essex, Myron, 27
Eu, Geoffrey, 24
Evans, H., 117
Evans, J., 115
Ewald, Paul W., 154, 162
Ewing, William E., 90,
Eyster, M.E., 116

Falick, Russel, 146
Fallopius, Gabriel, 132
Fan, P.T., 24, 163

Farid, B.T., 148
Farmer, John S., 131, 143
Farmer, Paul, 12, 13, 26
Fauci, Anthony, 68
Feiner, C., 143
Feldman, Douglas A., 64
Feldschuh, Joseph, 60
Fettner, Ann Giudici, 25
Fiddle, Seymour, 89
Fields, Bernard N., 27, 162
Finlayson, R., 63
Fischl, M.A., 115, 119
Fishbein, Martin, 124, 142
Fitzgerald, Frances, 88
Fitzpatrick, James K., 60
Flaskerud, Jacquelyn, 145
Fletcher, Mary Ann, 80n., 89, 115
Flowers, John V., 142
Fong, Geoffrey T., 142
Forney, Mary Ann, 146
Fox, Robin, 61, 63
Fraioli, Deborah, 65
Francis, Donald P., 61, 64, 115, 143
Fransen, Lieve, 121
Freeman, Linda, 147
Freitas, R., 121
Frevens, Pierre, 119
Friedland, Gerald H., 65, 117
Friedman, Samuel R., 64, 143, 148
Froland, S.S., 26
Fry, P., 121
Fuchs, E.J., 63
Fullilove, Mindy Thompson, 90, 91, 118, 144, 146
Fullilove, Robert E., 90, 91, 118, 146
Furtado, Ken, 142

Gaidusek, D.C., 27
Gail, M.H., 116
Gakinya, M.N., 117
Gallo, Robert C., 116, 119
Galvan, U., 143
Gardner, M., 27
Gardner, Pierce, 62
Garrett, Gerald R., 89
Garry, R.F., 26
Gear, A.J., 27
Gear, J.H.S., 27
Gear, J.S.S., 27

Gebbie, Christine, 139
Gharakhanian, S., 119
Giannattasio, Emily, 65
Gibson, David R., 144
Gilbert, Louisa, 145
Giliary, T., 26
Gilman, Alfred, 62
Ginzburg, Harold M. 60, 144
Girardi, E., 119
Gitlin, Todd, 61
Glass, Sarah, 115, 143
Goedert, J.J., 116
Gold, Mark S., 91
Goldberg, Martin, 91, 146
Golden, Jeffrey A., 24
Goldman, R., 63
Goldsby, Richard, 60
Goldstein, Marjorie F., 148
Goldstein, Paul J., 89, 91, 117
Gollub, Erica L., 146
Gomma, M., 143
Gomperts, E.D., 27
Gonzaga, A., 60
Goodman, Louis S., 62
Gopalakrishna, K.V., 116
Gordis, Enoch, 62
Gostin, Larry, 89
Gottfreid, Robert S., 21, 28
Gottlieb, A., 26
Gottlieb, M.S., 24, 26, 163
Goudsmit, J., 27
Gould, Peter, 120, 162
Grady, William R., 119
Grant, Charisse L., 90
Grant, R., 61
Greene, J.B., 24, 163
Greenfield, Lawrence, 89
Gregerson, Edgar, 120
Greve, Frank, 90
Griffin, James, 80n., 89
Grimes, J., 145
Grinspoon, Lester, 91, 118
Grmek, Mirko D., viii, 12, 25, 26, 155, 162
Gromyko, Alexander, 61
Grose, Francis, 132, 144
Gross, J., 117
Gross, Robert E., 118
Gross, Shirley A., 91, 146
Grund, Jean-Paul C., 64, 148
Gueguen, M., 116

Guerra, Solon C., 24
Guillebaud, John, 146
Guimaraes, C.D., 121
Guinan, M.E., 91
Guyader, Mireille, 27
Guydish, Joseph R., 144

Hadler, Stephen C., 62
Hagan, H., 147
Hamed, Ansley, 90
Hammershlak, N., 60
Handley, Margaret A., 144
Handsfield, H. Hunter, 25
Hankins, A., 144
Hansen, Gerhard, 156n.
Hanson, Bill, 89
Hardy, Daniel B., 122
Harris, Carol, 64
Harris, J.R.W., 116
Harrison, C., 143
Hart, G.J., 147
Hartgers, C., 147
Hassig, Susan, 121, 144
Hauer, L.B., 115
Haverkos, Harry W., 45, 62, 105, 117, 119
Haymann, David L., 61
Hays, Robert B., 148
Hearst, Norman, 115, 144
Heide, Kathleen M., 145
Hellman, Samuel, 25, 26, 27, 61, 119
Helms, Jesse, 157
Henig, Robin Marantz, 2n., 25, 162
Henley, William E., 131n., 143
Henriques, Fernando, 88, 120
Hernandez-Avila, Mauricio, 147
Hersh, Bradley H., 61
Hersh, Evan M., 62
Hessol, N.A., 119
Heyl, B.S., 117
Hildebrandt, Deborah A., 90, 118
Hilliard, Bobby, 144
Hilts, Philip J., 90
Hirsch, M.S., 115
Ho, D.D., 60
Hoegsberg, B., 118
Hoff, Colleen, 142
Hofstadter, Richard, 16, 26
Holmberg, S.D., 115
Holmes, King K., 18n., 62, 121, 146
Holzman, R.T., 24, 163

Hood, Harold V., 142
Hooker, M., 115., 116
Hopkins, William, 143
Hornblower, Margot, 120
Horsburg, C.R., 115
Howard, L., 116
Howard, S., 115
Howells, J., 116
Htop, M., 91
Hudson, Rock, 22
Huet, Thierry, 27
Hughes, W.T., 24
Huisman, J., 64
Hulley, Stephen, 144
Huminer, D., 26
Hunter, Tricia L., 146
Hutchinson, E.P., 60
Hymes, Kenneth B., 64

Inciardi, James A., 62, 63, 64, 80n. 84n., 89, 90, 117, 118, 120, 122, 143, 145
Issacson, M., 27
Itri, Vincenza, 119
Iverson, Annette E., 142

Jacobson, Lisa, 144
Jaffe, Harold W., 25, 61, 90, 115, 118, 122
Janot, C., 116
Jeffries, D.J., 116
Jemmott, John B., 142
Jemmott, Loretta S., 142
Jennings, A., 116
Jenum, P., 26
Jewell, L.D., 26
Jewell, N.P., 116
Jezek, Zdenek, 61
Jimenez, Antonio D., 89
Johnson, A.M., 115, 116, 147
Johnson, B.K., 27
Johnson, Bruce D., 89
Johnson, Thomas, 64
Johnson, Wendell A., 89
Jones, J.P. 64
Jose, Benny, 148
Joseph, Jill G., 142
Judson, Franklyn N., 62, 145

Kalichman, Seth C., 146
Kanchanaraksa, Sukon, 61

Kane, Normie, 89
Kanki, Phyllis J., 26, 27
Kanvamupira, Jean-Baptiste, 119
Kaplan, Barbara J., 146
Kaplan, C.D., 64
Kaplan, Edward, 147
Kaplan, John, 63
Kaposi, Moritz, 4
Karasira, P., 117
Karkham, P.D., 63
Kaslow, Richard A., 61, 64, 115
Katner, H.P., 26
Kean, B.H., 5, 25
Keet, I.P.M., 119
Kegeles, M., 148
Kegeles, Susan, 144
Kelly, Jeffrey A., 142, 146
Kennedy, John F., 16, 20
Kennedy, Robert F., 16n., 20
Kenny, C., 116
Kerr, P., 118
Kesey, Ken, 20
Kew, M.C., 27
Khoshnood, Kaveh, 147
Khoury, Elizabeth L., 143
Kingsley, Lawrence A., 144
Kinsella, James, viii, 28, 65
Kinsie, P.M., 117
Kippax, Susan, 148
Klein, Robert S., 65, 117
Klepinger, Daniel H., 119
Klimas, N., 115
Koch, Gary G. 143
Koech, Davy, 116, 121
Koester, S., 64
Kok, G.J., 144, 148
Kolata, Gina, 142
Koop, C. Everett, 125n.
Koornhof, H.J., 27
Korber, Bette, 162
Kovacs, Joseph A., 25
Kramer, Larry, 9n, 22, 28, 59, 68-70, 88
Krasinski, Keith, 119, 143
Kreiss, J.K., 116, 117
Kreiss, Joan J., 121
Kuhns, Joseph B. 145
Kunimoto, D., 26

Laa, Marie, 144
Laga, Marie, 115, 116, 121, 162

L'Age-Stehr, J., 116
Lamar, J.V., 117
Lambert, T., 116
Landesman, S., 118
Landis, Suzanne E., 143
Lang, W., 61, 63
Lange, M., 24, 163
Langmuir, A.D., 162
Larson, Ann, 121
Laughton, Barbara, 61
Lawlor, J., 117
Lazzarin, Adriano, 116
Leake, Barbara, 145
LeCharpentier, Y., 25
Leeper, Mary Ann, 146, 147
Lefrere, J.J., 116
Leibowitch, Jacques, viii
Leigh, Barbara C., 119
Leishman, K., 122
Leonard, Jonathan, 24
Letvin, N.L., 27
Levens, D., 26
Levine, Brian, 145
Levine, Martin P., 88
Levy, Jay A., 24, 61, 115
Lewis, B.J., 24
Lewis, Charles, 145
Lewis, Elaine, 120
Lewis, Nancy, 91, 122
Lewis, Paul, 120
Leyland, Winston, 61
Li, Ling, 146
Li, X.L., 60
Lidz, Charles W., 89
Lieb, Spencer, 122
Lifson, A.R., 119
Lightfoote, Marilyn, 122
Lindboe, C.F., 26
Linnestad, P.J., 26
Lipshutz, C., 143
Lipton, Douglas S., 89
Lloyd, G., 116
Lockwood, Dorothy, 64, 84n., 118
Louria, Donald B., 62
Lsokoski, S.L., 63
Luby, J.P., 27
Luciw, P.A., 27
Lyman, D.M., 61, 62, 63

Ma, Pearl, 25, 115, 119
Maas, Lawrence, 9n., 59

MacDonald, Mhairi G., 60
MacDonald, Patrick T., 91
MacInnes, Kersti, 162
Maclean, P., 63
Magana, J.R., 119
Maitha, G.M., 117
Malthus, Thomas Robert, 29, 30, 31
Manchester, William, 61
Mandel, G.L., 24
Mann, Jonathan M., 60
Manning, A., 143
Mansel, Peter W.A., 62
Maplethorpe, Robert, 43n.
Mardh, Per-Anders, 18n., 62
Marianetti, Mercia M.M., 24
Marin, Barbara, 144
Marko, Jim, 88
Marmor, M., 143
Marquis, L., 115, 145
Martin, G.S., 143
Martin, John L., 46, 62
Martin, L.S., 63
Martinez, Anthony, 24
Martinez, Samuel A., 56, 57, 64
Martini, G.A., 27
Mash, Deborah C., 63, 90
Masur, Henry, 24, 25, 163
Matusow, Allen J., 61
Mayimona, Kivuvu, 121, 144
Maynard, James E., 62
McBride, Duane C., 63, 64, 80n., 89,
   90, 122, 143
McCarthy, Joseph, 16
McCoy, Alfred, 120
McCoy, Clyde B., 63, 80n., 89, 90, 118,
   122, 143
McCoy, H. Virginia, 63, 80n., 89, 118,
   122, 143, 145
McDougal, J.S., 63
McElrath, Karen, 118
McGuire, Gerilyn, 65
McKenna, Neil, 120
McKitrick, John C., 65
McLean, K.A., 116
McNeill, James H., 28
McNeill, William H., 21, 162
Meese, Edwin, 160
Meilke, B.W., 26
Menezes, Carlos A.S., 24
Meyerhans, Andreas, 27
Meyers, A.M., 27

Michaelis, B., 115
Michelis, M.A., 24, 163
Mildvan, Donna, 64
Miles, Christine, 118
Miller, D.L., 116
Miller, E.M., 117
Miller, G.B., 27
Miller, Heather G., 143
Miller, James, 69, 88
Miller, Thomas, 89
Miller, Timothy E., 142
Miner, Richard C., 147
Minkoff, H., 118
Mirin, Steven M., 91, 118
Misztal, B.A., 121
Modigliani, R., 25
Mohr, Richard D., 43n.
Mokwa, K., 121, 144
Moll, Bernice, 64
Moody, H., 117
Moore, Joseph N., 62
Morand, Paul, 88
Moreau, Ron, 120
Morgante, S., 143
Morris, Charles R., 61
Morris, Lloyd, 88
Moses, Lincoln E., 143
Moss, A.R., 143
Moss, D., 121
Moss, V., 116
Most, H., 63
Motyl, Mary R., 65
Moudgil, T., 60
Mugerwa, R.D., 20n.
Murphy, Brian R., 162
Murphy, Frederick A., 27
Murphy, Sheigla, 89, 91
Murphy, Timothy F., 88
Murray, H.W., 24, 163
Musicco, Massimo, 116
Myers, Gerald, 162

Nahlen, Bernard L., 56, 57, 64
Narain, J.P., 121
Narciso, N., 119
Narkunas, John P., 122
Ndinya-Achola, J.O., 117, 121
Neaigus, Alan, 148
Nelson, Ann, 121, 144
Nelson, L., 145
Newell, Guy R., 62

Ngugi, Elizabeth N., 117, 121
Nickerson, Mark, 62
Nicod, A., 116
Nicolosi, Alfredo, 116
Norman, Colin, 122
North, M.L., 116
Nottingham, J., 27
Nsanze, Herbert, 121
Nugeyre, M.T., 63
Nwanyanwu, Okey C., 56, 57, 64
Nyamathi, Adeline, 145
Nyland, Thomas, 62
Nzabihimana, Elie, 119
Nzila, Nzilambi, 121, 144

O'Brien, Thomas R., 143
O'Donnell, John A., 64
Offermann, G., 116
O'Hanlon, Redmond, 24
O'Keefe, Elaine, 147
O'Malley, P.M., 119
Onions, C.T., 144
Onorato, I., 24, 163
Osborne, L., 115, 116
Osmond, D., 117
Ostrow, David G., 62
Ouellet, Lawrence J., 89
Oxtoby, Margaret J., 61
Oyafuso, L., 60

Padian, Nancy S., 61, 62, 63, 115, 116,
   143, 145
Page, J. Bryan, 63, 64, 80n., 89, 90
Pankey, G.A., 26
Paolino, Anna Maira, 119
Pappas, L., 147
Parker, John, 138
Parker, Richard G., 61, 121
Parks, W., 115
Parmet, Wendy E., 162
Parry, J.V., 147
Partridge, Eric, 144
Pearce, R.B., 63
Peck, David F., 146
Peterman, T.A., 115
Peterson, E., 162
Peterson, John, 144
Petherick, A., 115, 116
Petrow, Steven, 48, 63
Phair, John, 61
Picano, Felice, 62, 89

Piel, Jonathan, 26, 60
Pinching, A.J., 116
Piot, Peter, 60, 115, 116, 117, 121, 144
Pitlik, S.D., 26
Plant, Martin A., 146
Plant, Moria L., 146
Plummer, F.A., 116, 117, 121
Poirier, Suzanne, 88
Polk, B. Frank, 61, 119
Pomeroy, K.L., 27
Popovici, Florin, 61
Pottieger, Anne E., 84n., 118
Potts, Malcolm, 144
Preble, Edward, 89
Proctor, Donna, 145
Puro, V., 119
Pyle, G.F., 116

Quinlan, Judith A., 64
Quinn, Thomas C., 60, 61, 62, 121

Radetsky, Peter, 162
Ragni, M.V., 116
Rangel, Charles, 139
Rather, Dan, 22, 49
Ratner, Mitchell S., 90, 91, 118
Ray, G.G., 162
Raymond, C.A., 147
Reagan, Nancy, 22, 160, 163
Reagan, Ronald, 22, 159-160, 163
Reckless, Walter, 88
Redfield, R.R., 117
Reed, David L., 145
Reichert, C., 26
Reid, T., 147
Reinarman, Craig, 91
Resnick, L.K., 63, 90
Rettig, Richard P., 89
Reuben, James M., 62
Reynolds, Gladys, 62
Rezza, G., 143
Ribble, D.J., 143
Riggs, J., 61
Rinalso, Charles, 61
Rivers, James E., 63, 90, 143
Rizzetto, A., 143
Robert-Guroff, Marjorie, 116, 119
Roberts, Pacita, 121
Robertson, R., 115, 116
Robilotti, J.G., 63
Rodden, Pam, 148

Rodrigues, L., 120
Roelants, Georges, 27
Rogan, E., 26
Rolfs, Robert T., 91, 146
Rompalo, Anne, 25
Ronald, Allan R., 121
Roosevelt, Franklin D., 16
Root-Bernstein, Robert, 62
Rosenbaum, Marsha, 117, 118
Rosenberg, Ethel, 16
Rosenberg, Julius, 16
Rosenberg, Michael J. 145, 146
Rosenberg, Steven A., 25, 26, 27, 61, 119
Royko, Mike, 8
Rozenbaum, W., 119
Rullan, John V., 56, 57, 64
Rutherford, George W., 61, 63, 119
Rutledge, J.H., 143
Rutledge, Leigh W., 25, 61, 88, 163
Ryder, Robert W., 121, 144

Sacco, William P., 145
Sadigursky, Moises, 24
St. Lawrence, Janet S., 142
Sakondhavat, C., 147
Salahuddin, S., 63
Saltzman, Brian R., 65
Samuel, M.C., 61,143
Sanchez, M., 143
Sande, M.A., 117
Sanders, C.V., 27
Sandfort, T.G.M., 119, 144, 148
Sanger, William W., 88, 120
Sante, Luc, 88
Saphier, N., 143
Saracco, Alberto, 116
Sato, P.A., 60
Saxon, A., 24, 163
Schanker, H., 24, 163
Schilling, Robert F., 145, 147
Schmeidler, James, 89
Schneider, R., 27
Schoenthal, Rhea, 120
Schooley, R.T., 115
Schreeder, Marshall T., 62
Schroff, R., 24, 163
Schultz, S., 91
Schwartz, A., 116
Scott, G.B., 91
Seidlin, Mindell, 119

Selvin, Molly, 18n.
Selwyn, P.A., 143
Serpelloni, G., 143
Serwadda, D., 20n.
Setters, Jo, 146
Sewankambo, N.K., 20n.
Seymour, Richard, 62
Shah, Syed M., 63, 90
Shannon, G.W., 116, 117
Shapshak, Paul, 63, 90
Sharrar, Robert G., 91, 146
Shayne, Vivian T., 146
Sher, R., 27
Shergold, C., 116
Sherlock, Italo, 24
Shiboski, S.C., 116
Shilts, Randy, viii, 6, 11, 11n., 24-25, 28, 59, 70, 88
Shine, Daniel, 64
Shively, Charley, 39-40, 61
Short, Roger V., 144
Sibomana, J., 116
Siegal, Frederick P., 12, 25
Siegal, Harvey A., 146
Siegal, Marta, 12, 25
Siegel, David, 144
Siegert, R., 27
Silverstein, Charles, 62, 89
Simmons, Ann M., 120
Simms, Claudia, 120
Simons, Marlise, 120
Simonsen, J.N., 116, 117
Sing, T., 91
Slamon, D.J., 60
Small, Butkus, 64
Smilovici, W., 116
Smith, D.H., 27
Smith, David E., 62
Smith, Prince C., 89
Sohn, N., 63
Solomon, J., 162
Sonigo, Pierre, 27
Sonnett, H., 26
Sonnex, C., 115, 116
Sorensen, James L., 144
Sotheran, J., 143
Sparling, P. Frederick, 18n., 62
Spears, Richard A., 131n.
Spigland, Ilya, 64
Spitz, Margaret R., 62
Spitzer, P.G., 119

Spunt, Barry, 89
Stahl, Rosalyn E., 25, 64
Stalin, Joseph, 16
Stall, Ron D., 142
Steele, Fintan R., 60, 115
Steele, Stuart, 146
Stein, Zena A., 146
Stephen, B.H., 115
Stephens, Richard C., 64
Sterk, Claire, 91
Stewart, Laura, 146
Stier, Ken, 120
Stimson, G.V., 142, 147
Stone, Oliver, 16
Stoneburner, Rand, 64, 90, 115, 118
Strickler, R.B., 24
Strug, David, 64
Suffredini, Anthony F., 24
Sununu, John, 68

Taelman, H., 26, 115, 116
Tanfer, Koray, 119
Tarleton, Thomas, 120
Tchamouroff, S., 115, 116
Tealman, H., 117
Telzak, Edward E., 90, 117
Temple, Mark T., 119
Terry, P., 116
Thiam, Manoka Abib, 121, 144
Thomas, Charles C., 118
Thompson, Karla, 145
Thompson, Sumner E., 62
Thompson, Warren, 60
Tiollais, Pierre, 27
Tondo, M., 60
Tondreau, S., 63
Torres, Manual J., 89
Touchette, Nancy, 28
Trapido, Edward, 63, 80n., 89, 90, 91, 122, 143
Trappler, B., 27
Treaster, Joseph B., 90
Trocki, Karen F., 119
Tross, S., 118
Truman, Harry S., 16
Turner, Charles F., 143
Turshen, Meredeth, 122
Tyler, Patrice, 65
Tyrell, D.J., 26

Underhill, G.S., 116

Valdiserri, Ronald O., 145
Valentine, Fred, 119
van den Hoek, Johanna A.R., 148
Van de Perre, Phillipe, 116, 119
Van der Stuyft, Patrick, 116
Van der Walls, F.W., 27
Vande Stouwe, R.A., 24, 163
Van Dyck, Eddy, 121, 144
van Griensven, Godfried J.P. 119, 144, 148
van Lent, N.A., 119
Van Santen, G.W., 147
Vercauteren, Gaby, 115, 116
Veren, S.Z., 63
Verster, A.D., 147
Viorst, Milton, 61
Visco, G., 119
Visscher, Barbara R., 61, 144
Vittecoq, D., 116
Voeller, Bruce, 146
Vogt, M.W., 115
Volberding, P.A., 24, 117
Volinn, Ilse J., 157
Voth, A., 26

Wain-Hobson, Simon, 27
Waiyaki, P., 117
Waldorf, Dan, 89, 91
Walker, Andrew L., 89
Wallace, Barbara C., 90
Wallace, Joyce, 119
Wallace, Lew, 156, 162
Walters, James M., 89
Wang, Jichuan, 146
Ward, J.W., 115
Ward, Thomas P., 148
Washton, Arnold M., 91
Waters, W., 142
Watters, John K., 143
Weatherby, Norman L., 63, 90
Webster, Robert G., 162

Wefring, K.W., 26
Weinberg, Martin S., 88
Weiner, Jodie, M., 145
Weiner, N.J., 119
Weismal, J.D., 24, 163
Weiss, L., 143
Weiss, Phillip, 88
Weiss, Roger D., 91, 118
Weiss, Stanley H., 64
Weissman, Gloria, 144
Welsing, Frances Cress, 18, 27
Wermuth, Laurie A., 144
Wiebel, W. Wayne, 64, 89
Wiesner, Paul J., 18n., 62
Wiley, J.A., 61, 115, 143
Williams, Colin J., 88
Williams, P., 147
Williams, Terry, 90
Winick, Charles, 117
Winkelstein, W., 61, 62, 63, 115
Wish, Eric, 64
Witt, D.J., 115
Witte, C.L., 26
Witte, John J., 122
Witte, M.H., 26
Wofsey, C.B., 115, 117
Wolf, R.A., 24, 163
Woodward, N., 147
Wormser, Gary P., 24, 25, 64, 142, 163
Worth, Dooley, 145, 146
Worthen, T.D., 162
Wrong, Dennis, 60

Yancovitz, Stanley R., 64
Young, Douglas B., 157n.

Zacarais, R.K., 121
Zaccarelli, M., 119
Zolotusca, Laurentiu, 61
Zweig, M., 91

Subject Index

A

ACIDS (Acquired Community Immune Deficiency Syndrome), 6
Acquired Immune Deficiency Syndrome. *See* AIDS
ACT UP (the AIDS Coalition to Unleash Power), 60
Advocate, The, 58
Africa
    AIDS in, 1, 13-15, 32, 34, 35
    AIDS conspiracies and, 18-20
    AIDS origin, 153-155
    HIV transmission in, 33-35, 155
African green monkey, 14, 18, 20, 154
AIDS
    acceleration of, 150-152
    acronyms for, 5-6
    beginnings, 3-8, 13-15
    behavioral problem, 124-125
    Bush administration and, 160
    clinical studies, 22
    conspiracies, 16-20
    definition, vi, 10
    education, 125-127
    epidemiology of, 31-38, 150-152
    exponential growth rate, 31
    future of, 153-155
    in Haiti, 12-13, 14, 33-35
    "Haitian connection," 12
    incubation period, 48, 152
    infectious etiology for, 8
    Kaposi's sarcoma and, 3, 4, 9, 11, 45, 47, 54-55
    media, and, 21-23, 58-59
    mortality rate, 14, 152
    onset of, 48
    origin of, 153, 155
    pediatric, 15, 33, 36-37
    Pneumocystis carinii pneumonia (PCP) and, 3, 9, 54
    quarantine, 156-159
    Reagan administration and, 22-23, 68, 125n., 159-160
    research, 22, 161
    "risk-groups," 12, 93
    symptoms of, vi
    vaccines, 123-124, 161
    See also HIV
"AIDS Czar," 139
AIDS prevention/risk reduction
    behavioral problem, 124-125, 161
    condoms, female, 133-137
    condoms, male, 131-132
    condom use, 141
    education, AIDS, 125-127, 161
    injection drug users and, 127-131
    Miami NADR project, 129-131
    National AIDS Demonstration Research (NADR), 129
    needle exchange programs, 137-140
    outreach workers, 129, 130
    prevention messages, 161
    research, 161
    risk reduction programs, 126-127, 161
    risk reduction programs, culturally appropriate, 128-131
    risk reduction programs, for women 133-137
    safer sexual practices, 129
    sterile injection equipment, 129
    vaccines, 161
AIDS transmission. *See* HIV transmission
Alan Guttmacher Institute, 152
Alcohol, HIV transmission cofactor, 43, 45
Amebiasis, 47
American Foundation for AIDS Research, 22
Amebic dysentery, 2
Amphetamines, 74
Amyl nitrite, 7, 43-45
Anal intercourse, 6, 40-47, 71-73, 94, 112
Anal warts, 6, 47

Antiparasitic drugs, 47
Asia, AIDS in, 32, 35
Australia, AIDS in, 32-33

B

Bacillary dysentery, 2
Bathhouses, gay, 39, 70-73
Battelle Memorial Institute, 106
Behavioral research, AIDS preven-
    tion, 161
Belle Glade, Florida, 113-114
Bisexual HIV transmission, 32, 36
Black Death, 149, 151
Black Death, The, 21
Blackwater fever, 2
Blade, 58
Blood bank industry, 158-159
Blood/blood products
    HIV transmission vector, 9, 10, 33,
        35, 37
    injection drug users exchange of,
        50, 53, 78, 79
    testing, 33, 160
Blood transfusion patients, 8, 9
Booting/jacking, 50, 53, 78, 79
Boston AIDS brigade, 138
Brazil, AIDS in, 110-112
Burundi, 13, 19
Bush administration, 139, 160
Butyl nitrite, 7, 43-45

C

CAIDS (Community Acquired Im-
    mune Deficiency Syndrome), 6
California Partners Study, 96
Canada, AIDS in, 32-33
Centers for Disease Control
    AIDS acronyms and, 5
    AIDS prevention messages, 161
    AIDS tracking, 8, 9, 35
    Belle Glade, Florida, study, 113
    heterosexual AIDS cases, 93
    injection drug users AIDS cases, 49
    needle exchange programs and,
        139-140
    "patient zero," search for, 10
    PCP, first reports of, 3
    "wasting syndrome" cases, 55
Central nervous system complica-
    tions, HIV tertiary stage, 48
Chagas' disease, 2

Chancroid, 152
Clinton administration, 139
Cocaine, 74, 76, 78, 82
Condoms
    AIDS prevention and, 161
    in bathhouses, 73
    education, 74
    female, 132-137
    HIV transmission prevention, 131-
        137
    male, 131-132
    prostitution and, 106, 133, 134,
        158
    in sex clubs, 74
    subcultural issue, 127
Congenital immune deficiency, 5
Conspiracies, AIDS, 16-20
Cookers (injection equipment), 51
Copping, 74
Cottons (injection equipment), 51
Crack, sex for
    in crack houses, 83
    data, 84-85
    HIV infection and, 84, 86, 87
    pharmacological, 85-86
    sociocultural, 85, 86
    See also HIV transmission, crack
        related
Crack, sexually transmitted diseases
    and, 86-87, 100-102
Crack-cocaine, 82-83
Crack houses, 83
Cryptococcosis, 54-55
Cryptosporidiosis, 5
Cryptosporidium parasite, 5

D

Dade County Stockade, Miami, 52
Dengue fever, 2
Department of Health and Human
    Services, 125
Diarrhea, HIV tertiary stage, 48
Drug abuse treatment, AIDS preven-
    tion, 161
Drug users. See Injection drug users
Drug use/sexual risk analysis, 45-46

E

Eastern Europe, AIDS in, 35-36
Ebola fever, 1, 2
EIA (HIV test), 10

ELISA (enzyme-linked immunosorbent assay), 10
Epidemiology of AIDS, 31-38
Essay on the Principle of Population, An, 29

F

Faggots, 69, 70
Fever, high, HIV tertiary stage, 48
Fisting, 43, 70
"Four-H Club," 12

G

Gay activists, 23
"Gay bowel syndrome," 6, 40
"Gay cancer," 11, 150
Gay community, 58, 69, 126
Gay Community News, 58
"Gay compromise syndrome," 6n.
Gay liberation, 6, 39
Gay Liberation Front, 39
Gay Men's Health Crisis, 69
"Gay plague," 8, 93, 150
Gay Power, 58
Gay press, 58-59
Gay rights ordinance, 7, 8
Gay sex scene
  bathhouses, 39, 70-73
  commercialization of, 71
  condoms, 73, 74
  ethnographic study of, 71-73
  Faggots, 69
  fisting, 43, 70
  "J.O." (jack-off) clubs, 74
  rimming, 7, 47
  safe sex messages, 73
  sex, anal, 6, 40-47, 72
  sex clubs, 73-74, 87
  sex, high-risk, 71
  sex, oral, 72
  See also HIV transmission, homosexual
Genital herpes, 6
Genital warts, 47
Giardiasis, 47
Gonorrhea, 6, 40, 47, 102, 152
GRID (Gay-Related Immune Deficiency), 5-6, 93

H

Haiti

AIDS in, 12-13, 14, 33-35
AIDS growth rate in, 33-35
cryptosporidiosis epidemic in, 5
opportunistic infections in, 4-5
"risk group," 11-12, 35
"Haitian connection," 12
Hantavirus Pulmonary Syndrome (HPS), 153
Hemophiliacs, 8, 9
Hepatitis B, 6, 71
Heroin, 74, 76, 77, 78
Heterosexual HIV transmission. *See* HIV transmission, heterosexual
HIV (human immunodeficiency virus)
  definition, vii, 10
  identification of, 9
  infection manifestations, 54-57
  stages of, 48-49
  test (EIA), 10
  vaccines, 123-124, 150
HIV-1, 10n.
HIV-2, 10n., 154
HIV infection manifestations, injection drug users, 54-57
HIV infection stages, homosexual men, 48-49
HIV transmission
  bisexual, 32, 36
  blood/blood products, contact with, 9, 10, 33, 35, 37
  body fluids, exchange of, 10
  "bridging groups,", 41, 93, 95
  crack and, 82. *See also* HIV transmission, crack related; Crack, sex for
  future of, 153-155
  health care and, 34, 35
  heterosexual, 93
  homosexual, 38-40
  injection drug users, 49-50
  mother to child (perinatal), 10, 33, 34
  prevention, 155
  prostitutes and, 34, 35
  sexually transmitted diseases and, 35, 152
  women and, 33, 110, 132, 133-137, 152
HIV transmission, crack-related
  anal sex and, 104

condom use and, 103, 104
female-to-male, 102
hypersexuality and, 83, 84, 102-103
immune systems and, 103
male sexual response, 84
male-to-female, 102
male-to-male, 104
multiple partners, 84, 85, 87, 102
pharmacological, 85-86, 103
oral sex and, 104-105
sexually transmitted diseases and, 86, 103
socio-cultural, 85, 86
vaginal sex and, 104
See also Crack, sex for
HIV transmission, heterosexual, viii
in Africa, 98, 99, 112
AIDS bridge, 95
AIDS epidemiology and, 32-33, 34, 35, 38
anal intercourse and, 94
bisexual partners and, 93
blood as HIV vector, 97
bridge to, 41
California Partners' Study, 96
cofactors of, 96
condom use, 97, 98
female-to-male, 94, 97-99
frequency of contact, 97
Haitians and, 93
hemophiliacs, 93
injection drug user partners, 93
Italian Study Group on HIV Heterosexual Transmission, 97
male-to-female, 94, 96-97
seropositive partner, 96, 97
semen as HIV vector, 94, 97
sex for crack. *See* HIV transmission, crack related; crack, sex for
sexually transmitted diseases and, 94, 97, 98, 100-102
in the United States, 113-11
vaginal secretions as HIV vector, 94
See also Prostitution
HIV transmission, homosexual
alcohol and, 43, 45
anal intercourse and, 6, 40-47
blood as HIV vector, 40

"bridge" to heterosexuals, 41
cocaine and, 43, 46
contact with infected blood, 40
douching/enemas, 42, 43
enteric diseases, 6, 47
epidemiology of AIDS and, 32, 34, 35, 38
"fisting," 43
hepatitis B virus (HBV), 42
injection equipment, contaminated, 41
nitrite inhalants (amyl and butyl) and, 43
promiscuity and, 6, 39-40
rectal trauma and, 42
sex, oral-genital and, 41
sex partners, multiple/random, 6, 40-41, 45
sexually transmitted diseases (STD), 6, 47
See also Gay sex scene
HIV transmission, injection drug users
backloading and, 51, 52
blood as HIV vector, 50, 53, 78, 79
booting/jacking and, 50, 53, 78, 79
bridge group, 41
drawing up and, 52, 54
drug sharing and, 52
frontloading and, 51
"mainlining," 78
needle exchange programs, 137-140, 160, 161
needle rinsing and, 50
needle/syringe contamination study, 79-81
needle/syringe sharing and, 50, 54, 75, 78, 79
shooting back and, 52
tasters, 50, 76, 77
See also Shooting galleries
Homosexual men
enteric diseases and, 6, 47, 71
HIV infection cofactors and, 41-47
HIV infection stages in, 48-49
immunosuppression in, 3
Kaposi's sarcoma and, 3, 9
P. carinii pneumonia and, 3, 9
promiscuity and, 6, 39-40
sexually transmitted diseases (STD) and, 6, 47

See also Gay sex scene; HIV transmission, homosexual
Human immunodeficiency virus. *See* HIV
Human T-Cell Lymphotropic Virus, Type III (HTLV-III), 9

I

Immune deficiency, congenital, 5
Immune system dysfunction, antiparasitic drugs and, 47
  HIV and, vii
  KS connection, 4
  PCP connection, 3, 4
  unexplained, 5
Immunocompromised, 35
Immunosuppression, 3
Immunosuppressive drugs, 3
Infant HIV infection. *See* AIDS, pediatric, 15, 33, 36-37
Injection drug users
  AIDS etiology and, 8, 9, 32, 33
  cocaine, 51-52, 74, 76, 78
  copping, 53, 74
  dealers, 76, 77
  get off (inject drugs), 75
  heroin, 51, 52, 74, 76, 77, 78
  house doc, 77-78
  injection, methods of, 33n.
  injection equipment, 51, 75
  needle/syringe sharing, 75, 78, 79
  running partners (buddies), 53, 54, 76, 77
  "popping," 50
  risk reduction programs for, 127-131
  sex partners of, 9, 74
  speedball, 51
  tasters, 50, 76, 77
  "works," 52, 74
  See also HIV transmission, injection drug users; Shooting galleries
Institute for Survey Research, Temple University, 106
Institute of Tropical Medicine, Antwerp, 152
Institute of Tropical Medicine, Miami, 113
Intestinal parasites, 47

Intravenous drug users. *See* Injection drug users

J

"J.O." (jack-off) clubs, 74
Jackson Memorial Hospital, Miami, 4, 11, 49, 50

K

Kaposi's sarcoma (KS), 4, 9, 11, 45, 47, 54-55
  first reports, 3
  "gay cancer," 11
  in Haitians, 11
  immunosuppression and, 4
  injection drug users and, 54, 55
  intestinal parasites and, 47
  nitrite inhalants and, 45
  in non-AIDS populations, 4
  in Uganda, 4
Kenyatta Hospital, 34
Kisingani University, 14
Ku Klux Klan, 17

L

Latin American, 1, 32, 36
Legionnaire's disease, 57
Lymphadenophy-Associated Virus (LAV), 9

M

Macaques, 20
"Mainlining," 33n.
Malaria, 110
Malthus' theory, 29-31
Mandrills, 20
Marburg virus, 18-19
Methadone, 138
Mexico, AIDS in 32-33
Miami Community Outreach Study, 101
Middle East, 1, 35

N

NADR (National AIDS Demonstration Research), 101, 133
National Academy of Sciences, 124, 140
National AIDS Demonstration Research. *See* NADR
National Commission on AIDS, 124

National Institute of Allergy and Infectious Diseases, 105
National Institute on Drug Abuse, 45, 98, 100, 101, 133
National Institutes of Health
  HIV identification, 9
  HIV virus survival tests, 51
  nitrites and, 44
National Rifle Association, 17
Needle exchange programs, 137-140, 160, 161
Needles/syringes
  contamination study, 79-81
  rinsing, 50
  seropositive, 80, 81
  sharing, 50, 54
Neurological disorders, HIV infection tertiary stage, 48
New Haven's needle exchange program, 138
New York Gay Men's Health Project, 6
New York Native, 58
New Zealand, AIDS in, 32-33

O

Onchocerciasis ("river blindness"), 1, 2
One Flew Over the Cuckoo's Nest, 20
"Opportunistic" infections
  HIV infection tertiary stage, 48
  immune system dysfunction and, 4
  injection drug users and, 55
Oral sex, 71, 72, 103, 112

P

P. Carinni parasite, 3
Pasteur Institute, 3, 9, 51
"Patient Zero," 10-11
PCP. *See Pneumocystis carinii* (PCP)
Pediatric AIDS, 15, 33, 36-37
Perinatal HIV transmission, 10, 33, 34, 127
Pink Panthers, 38
The Plague, vii
Pneumocystis carinii (PCP), 3
  in Brazil, 3
  in guinea pigs, 3
  immunosuppression and, 3, 4
  injection drug users and, 50, 54
  in Paris, 3

"Poppers," 7, 43
"Popping" (drug injection), 33n.
Port-au-Prince Hospital, 12
Promiscuity, HIV infection cofactor, 6
Prostitution
  in Africa, 112
  AIDS link, 108
  in Brazil, 110-112
  condoms and, 106, 133, 134, 158
  drugs and, 108-110
  HIV infection studies of, 107
  HIV transmission and, 106-112
  in other countries, 107-108
  in Thailand, 108-110
  in the United States, 106-107

Q

Quarantine, AIDS, 157-158
Quarantine, behavioral, 158-159

R

Reagan administration and AIDS, 22-23, 68, 125n., 159-160
Respiratory complications, HIV infection tertiary stage, 48
Rimming, 7, 47
Risk reduction programs, 126-137, 161
Risk reduction programs for women, 133-137
"River blindness" (*onchocerciasis*), 1, 2
Rumania, 36-37
Rwanda, 19

S

SAIDS (Simian AIDS), 20
St. Louis City Hospital, 15
San Francisco AIDS Foundation, 48
San Francisco Men's Health Study, 42
Semen, HIV infection vector, 7
Seroconversion, 41n., 48
Seropositive, 80
Sex clubs, gay, 73-74
Sex for crack. *See* Crack, sex for
Sexual subculture, 111-112
Sexually transmitted diseases (STDs)
  crack and, 100-102
  HIV infection cofactor, 7, 35, 152
  homosexual men and, 6, 71

Shigella, 47
Shooting galleries
    blood exchange in, 78
    booting/jacking in, 78, 79
    cocaine and, 74, 76, 78
    copping and, 74
    get-off house, 75, 77
    getting off in, 74, 75
    heroin and, 74,
    injection kit and, 75
    "mainlining" in, 78
    needle rinsing in, 79
    needle/syringe sharing in, 75, 78, 79
    needle/syringe contamination study, 79-81
    running partners in, 76, 77
    sex partners in, 74
    tastes in, 50, 76, 77
    "works" in, 74, 76
Simian AIDS (SAIDS), 20
Simian immunodeficiency virus (SIV), 20, 154
"Slim" disease, 19n.
Smallpox, 157
"Snappers," 44
Sooty mangabeys, 20, 154
Soviet Academy of Sciences
Soviet Republic, AIDS in, 36
Spoons (injection equipment), 51
"Stonewall," 39
Stonewall Inn, 38
STOP AIDS program, 126-127
Sudan, 1-2
Survey of Chemical and Biological Warfare, 18
Syphilis, 6, 40, 47, 102, 152

T

T. gondii parasite, 4-5
Thailand, AIDS in, 108-110
Third International Conference on AIDS, 22
Toxoplasmosis, 4-5, 11, 54-55
Tuberculosis, 157
Tuskegee syphilis experiments, 18

TWIT, 58

U

Uganda, 4
Understanding Aids, 125
United States, AIDS in, 32, 38
U.S. National Cancer Institute, 13
University of Miami School of Medicine, 51, 101

V

Vaginal intercourse, 94, 106, 112
Vervet monkey, 18
Viral evolution, 153-155
Viral hemorrhagic fever, 18

W

Wasting, HIV infection tertiary stage, 48
"Wasting" disease, 19n.
"Wasting syndrome," 55, 56
Western Europe, AIDS in, 32-33
Wistar Institute in Philadelphia, 19
WOGS (Wrath of God Syndrome), 31n.
Women
    AIDS rate among, 33, 110, 132
    condom use and, 133-137
    female condom, 133-137
    HIV transmission and women, 133-137
    sexually transmitted diseases and, 152
World Health Organization
    African AIDS growth rate report, 32
    AIDS, worldwide, report on, 38
    AIDS conspiracies, and, 17-18
    AIDS in Rumania, report of, 37
    AIDS in Thailand, 108

Y

Yellow fever, 2, 157

Z

Zaire, 1, 13, 14, 15, 19